MeNoP

Awaken and Empower
your Self
with
Individualized Bio-Identical
Hormone Replacement Therapy

M.E. Ted Quigley, M.D.

Copyright 2015 by M.E. Ted Quigley

TABLE OF CONTENTS

Chapter 1

The Physician's Oath

I solemnly pledge to consecrate my life to the service of humanity.
I will give to my teachers the respect and gratitude that is their due.

I will practice my profession with conscience and dignity.

The health of my patient will be my first consideration.

I will respect the secrets that are confided in me, even after the patient has died.

I will maintain by all the means in my power, the honor and the noble traditions of the medical profession.

My colleagues will be my sisters and brothers.

I will not permit considerations of age, disease or disability, creed, ethnic origin, gender, nationality, political affiliation, race, sexual orientation, social standing or any other factor to intervene between my duty and my patient.

I will maintain the utmost respect for human life.

I will not use my medical knowledge to violate human rights and civil liberties, even under threat.

I make these promises solemnly, freely and upon my honor.

WHY I WROTE THIS BOOK

When I completed my medical training and took the Physician's Oath some 45 years ago, I swore to serve humanity, to practice medicine with conscience and dignity, and to maintain the utmost respect for human life. Those words have guided me through the years as a researcher and a physician. I have always known the health of my patients must be my first consideration, and that conviction has served as the backbone of my medical practice.

As a medical researcher, a Board Certified OB/GYN, and a Board Certified Reproductive Endocrinologist, I have had the privilege of witnessing the miracle of life time after time. I have delivered thousands of babies, so I have seen over and over again the incredible surge of intense unconditional love that is present when a newborn is held and nursed by her mother for the very first time. I have watched that surge of love intensify, as the maternal hormones increase during pregnancy and nature helps to ensure an unbreakable mother-child bond. But I have also seen how some new mothers experience intense emotional pain, suffering, and darkness after delivery, the result of rapidly plummeting hormones causing a hormonal deficiency.

My medical background and scientific training as a researcher have uniquely qualified me to be a neutral observer; I see how women are profoundly affected by the biological and hormonal changes in their bodies that happen throughout their lives, not only on a monthly basis, but also during pregnancy, and then again after the age of about 45, when the sex hormones responsible for reproduction begin to wane and most women begin the process of menopause. I have watched my patients through the years, as girls grow into mothers, and mothers grow into grandmothers, and have realized with a jolt that life's predictable transformations, from girl to woman, woman to mother, mother to grandmother, are all part of the same hormonal continuum.

YOUR HORMONES AFFECT YOU

Think back to those teenage years when your period first began, and you may remember being moody, with erratic behavior as your hormones first began the process of waking up your reproductive cycle. That moodiness, the tears and frustration of a girl becoming a woman are a result of the ever changing hormone levels revving up in the young girl/young woman's body.

Do you, or did you, suffer from PMS (Pre-Menstrual Syndrome)? If so, you are/were likely feeling moody, teary, frustrated, and angry. That's because every month your hormone levels fluctuate tremendously. Well, the same thing happens during menopause: your sex hormones fluctuate and wind down during the peri-menopause, eventually causing your monthly periods to cease at the menopause. Those familiar, erratic PMS issues later are accompanied with menopausal-related hot flashes, night sweats, migraines, depression, mood swings, memory loss, fatigue, reduced libido, and much more. In fact, you may have already experienced the menopause, so you know these symptoms can be significant. While some fortunate few women sail through menopause with few or no negative symptoms, others are tortured by terribly negative physical, mental, emotional, and/or cognitive changes.

HORMONE REPLACEMENT THERAPY

I am here to tell you there is a safe, scientifically proven approach to replace the hormones that begin their inevitable decline as you get older. I have used this method to treat thousands of women, helping to bring

3

back sanity and balance to their lives. It's called Individualized Bio-Identical Hormone Replacement Therapy, and includes replacing the female sex hormones Estrogen, Progesterone, and surprisingly, but importantly, the so called male sex hormone, Testosterone, which women also produce, although in much smaller amounts than men.

The use of hormone replacement therapy to treat menopausal symptoms in women has been around since World War II, when in 1942, the FDA approved Premarin, a form of estrogen extracted from pregnant mare's urine, and literally named for what it is; PREgnant MARe's urINe. From that time on, estrogen therapy became the cornerstone for managing menopausal symptoms, and to this day, clinicians and researchers still agree that the primary approach to treating menopausal symptoms is with estrogen replacement therapy. Things haven't changed all that much since 1942, because to this day Premarin, the estrogen pill made from pregnant mare's urine, is still the most widely prescribed form of estrogen replacement therapy, even though the non-oral, bio-identical estrogen patch, cream, or gel is, in my opinion, a safer and more effective option.

But conflicting information about estrogen replacement, which is often simply called hormone replacement, continues to be misreported in the news. One day, television news shows report hopefully that estrogen therapy can reduce the risk of heart attack after menopause. The next day, we hear that researchers have discovered evidence that estrogen therapy has once and for all been proven to increase the risk of breast cancer. Who's right? What if you are a breast cancer survivor experiencing severe menopausal symptoms? How does it affect you?

In my experience, too much conflicting information is often worse than no information at all. That's why it's critical to understand the scientific impact that the ovarian hormones such as estrogen, progesterone, and testosterone have on your body, mind, and well-being, and why maintaining healthy bio-identical levels of these vital sex hormones is so important for you to live a healthy, balanced, long life. In fact, by replacing and balancing these hormones, you may find that you'll make your life far more meaningful, productive, and enjoyable than you could ever imagine.

HOW THIS BOOK CAN HELP YOU

According to the National Institutes of Health, the average age when a woman in the United States experiences her last period is 51. And the World Health Organization reports that at age 60, the typical American woman today can expect to live an average of 24 additional years to age 84. This means that the average woman in the US will be post-menopausal for more than 30 years of her life.

Many women are surprised to learn that menopause is a uniquely human condition. In nature, few female animals outlive their reproductive capabilities, and actually, menopause in the human female is a relatively recent phenomenon. As late as 1900, the average life expectancy for a woman was just 47 years. Many women died during pregnancy, during delivery, or soon after (postpartum). With the discovery of antibiotics, improved obstetrical care, and better imaging and monitoring equipment, women now not only routinely survive pregnancy and delivery, they live far beyond the onset of menopause. In my own practice, I see patients who are healthy, active great-grandmothers.

This book describes a unique and proven method of bio-identical hormone replacement therapy that has been clearly shown in tens of thousands of women to counter the negative effects of menopause safely and effectively. My approach has been carefully developed over more than 35 years of medical research and clinical practice, of listening to my patients and making adjustments based on their feedback in order to bring balance back into their hormonal lives. It worked for them. It can work for you.

Menopause resulted in hot flashes and night sweats, frustration, a lack of patience, a problem focusing, a sense of "Is this all there is?" and a sadness that sexual life with "the love of my life"—my husband—was lacking fulfillment for both of us. After fine-tuning my estradiol and testosterone replacement to meet my needs by recording my daily progress on the Women's Awareness Calendar, I experienced a sense of calmness. This improved sense of well being has enabled me to give of myself, to everyone else in my life, and has allowed me to pursue my life's dream of helping others. Sex is great! Love is great! A peacefulness exists within me which allows me to see the good in each day, every person, and life. I love life! I see the bigger picture now. There is hope, and that hope is within you...you may need just a bit of assistance in accessing it. This is what the individualized, natural, biologically identical estrogen and testosterone hormone replacement did for me.

Nancy

REMEMBER!

Any program of hormone replacement takes time to work its wonders, and because we are all individuals, that time can be as short as hours, or as long as days or weeks. But my patients all see and feel the positive effects of bio-identical hormone replacement within just a few weeks time. With the proper dose of bio-identical hormone replacement you'll feel more energized too, and you'll feel more confident, less moody and depressed. Also, your libido will return and that will no doubt be a pleasant surprise for you and your spouse or partner. And you will look younger and feel better too. How? Estrogen increases collagen production, which softens and plumps the skin, helping to eliminate wrinkles. And by balancing your sex hormones, you'll find as your energy changes, so does your attitude. You'll just "feel" better as you're more balanced. Maintaining that balance means you may need to make some minor adjustments in dosages from time to time, but that's something you'll be able to personally control as you become more familiar with how your body responds to the replacement of each specific hormone.

I have personally treated more than 15,000 women over the years and each of them has proven to me that individualized bio-identical replacement of the sex hormones estrogen and testosterone—or estrogen and testosterone in combination with natural progesterone—will not only improve your quality of life, but may also increase your longevity and improve your overall outlook on life—safely and with very little risk of negative effects on your health.

KNOWLEDGE IS POWER AND EMPOWERMENT

The pages that follow are a one-stop source for information and self-evaluation relating to hormone replacement and its risks and benefits. In this book I provide you with information so that you'll be more aware of what might be happening to your body today and what is likely to happen to it tomorrow. I also describe the complete range of methods I prefer and why.

In addition, I share with you the Women's Awareness Calendar, a simple but essential tool that I have given to each of my patients since 1978 to chart changes in their health on a daily basis. The Women's Awareness Calendar is a great way to keep track of your PMS, Peri- menopausal or Menopausal symptoms and to understand what is working to keep you healthy and balanced. With it, you can monitor any changes occurring within your body, and discover for yourself whether you should consider hormone replacement therapy.

I know that as human beings, we are all so much more than the sum of our parts, and in my medical practice, my patients have shown me that a seemingly isolated problem or imbalance can affect the mind, body, emotion, and spirit as a whole. No one knows better than you what is going on with your body, what is right for you, and what you need to create a comfortable, even balance. I urge you to research your options, and then listen to your inner voice when it comes to taking control of your health and your life.

My goal in writing this book is to sweep away the years of misinformation that have been heaped on women over the past few decades about hormone replacement therapy, and clearly show you that individualized bio-identical sex hormone replacement therapy is not only safe, but it is something that every woman approaching menopause should seriously consider.

MENOPAUSE CAN BE AMAZING

The great news is that menopause, and the years post-menopause, can be the most amazing time of your life, giving you a better "you" than you ever could have imagined. First of all, you won't have a period to deal with every month. That's a huge plus for most women. And with a steady, even, balanced, flow of bio-identical estrogen, testosterone, and progesterone, you'll have the energy and the ability to follow your passion, and to re-discover your true Self.

I am both a doctor and researcher, so I know that Western science has come a long way in understanding the physical structure of the female body. I recognize that it has also progressed considerably in comprehending the relationships and inner workings of the mind. But in my nearly 45 years as a physician devoted primarily to women's health, I have discovered that there is a third component that is absent from Western medicine, one that must be addressed, recognized and respected when it comes to women: the mysterious, amazing wonder that is the female spirit.

I hope this book is the first step in your journey to recognizing the wondrous, unique spirit that is your true Self. I sincerely believe that the journey of self-discovery begins with balance. I know that by physically balancing your hormone levels, you are one step closer to emotional balance. That emotional balance can lead to empowerment. I have seen it happen thousands of times to thousands of women. I honestly believe that the light of the truth, in this case, the truth about hormone replacement therapy, will always prevail over the darkness of ignorance and misinformation.

It is my sincere hope that you let the words on these pages then be the light that helps you to discover your own truth, and the light that enables you to find your way to your intuitive true Self.

Chapter 2

Your Body, Hormones and You

A woman is the full circle.

Within her is the power to create, nurture, and transform.

Diane Mariechild

WHAT ARE HORMONES?

A hormone is a bio-chemical substance that is naturally created by a single organ, traveling throughout your entire body via your blood circulation to impact almost every cell in your body.

Hormones regulate many processes in the human body, from raising or lowering blood glucose levels with insulin and glucagon, to stimulating the production of milk with prolactin, to initiating the fight or flight response with epinephrine. The hormone estrogen is manufactured by and released primarily from your ovaries but, like all other hormones, it is then released into your circulatory system where it immediately travels throughout the entire body. As a result, estrogen impacts every cell in your body, including your bones, skin, brain, and heart, as well as your female organs.

Two major forms of estrogen are actually produced by the ovary: estradiol and estrone. Both of these estrogens are produced and released from the ovary 7 days a week, 24 hours a day, in varying amounts, throughout the menstrual cycle. And both of these more potent estrogens, estradiol and estrone, are eventually broken down or metabolized by the body into a much weaker form of estrogen called estriol.

HORMONES RULE REPRODUCTION

If you're a healthy woman between the ages of about 12 and 51, every month you'll get an important message from your body in the form of your period. A period means you're not pregnant, so if you're a healthy woman and your period doesn't come, there's a good chance that you are pregnant. Every woman knows this. Waiting for a period, hoping it will come or not come, is a uniquely female experience that is known, shared, and understood by women from every culture, country, and century.

But the biology that creates this experience is largely unknown or misunderstood by women, and unfortunately, sometimes by their doctors too.

The reality is, your cycle is simply a monthly ebb and flow of hormones that is carefully orchestrated by your body with one very important goal: the hope of creating a new life. But here's the catch. The amount of hormones released by your body, the kinds of hormones that are released, and the order and the timing of those hormones can have a dramatic effect on you. That means hormones affect your emotions, your physical and mental health, and your well being.

HORMONAL CONSISTENCY IS THE KEY

There are basically two times in life when the majority of women report that they are at their very best both emotionally and physiologically. Those are the times when their bodies either produce the greatest consistent amount of hormones, or perhaps surprisingly, the least.

Women who are pregnant and overflowing with hormones are said to glow. That glow isn't an illusion, it's very much a physiological reality, the result of consistently high levels of estrogen, progesterone, and testosterone released from the placenta during pregnancy. But that same quiet glow can also be seen in some grandmothers during their late post-menopausal years, when those same three hormones, estrogen, progesterone, and testosterone, are consistently at very low levels. The key word is consistently. When levels of hormones, whether high or low, are consistent, then feeling and being your very best is the natural result.

For menopausal women, this hormonal consistency can also be achieved using individualized bio-identical hormone replacement therapy. I have found that giving women a low, steady amount of each hormone each day can give my patients that same beautiful female glow that they may have experienced when they were pregnant.

But I have found that when their hormone levels fluctuate wildly, these same women can suffer wildly, with symptoms that manifest themselves physically, psychologically, emotionally, and spiritually. That's because an intensely steep drop or change in hormones, especially a drop in the hormone estrogen, can have a major physical impact on your entire body. If you've ever been pregnant, and delivered a child, you know exactly what I am saying, because the greatest estradiol crash a woman can ever experience occurs after childbirth, or postpartum. After delivering the baby and placenta, a mother's estradiol levels decline from 15,000 pg/ml to undetectable levels within just 48 hours. That's why many women experience intense emotions after their baby is born, and can often be seen laughing and crying literally at the same time. For most, it's a minor adjunct to the birth process; you may have heard it referred to as postpartum or post-baby blues. Fortunately, in most cases the effect of this estradiol crash usually disappears within a few days. But in its most severe form, postpartum depression can have a devastating impact on the woman, the newborn, and her family, and can sometimes last for months or even years. I believe this is the same kind of devastation caused by the hormone fluctuations of PMS (Pre-Menstrual-Syndrome), and by the hormone highs and lows of the Peri-Menopause and Menopause.

THE POWERFUL ESTROGEN CONNECTION

Every part of your body - your immune system, cardiovascular, respiratory, gastrointestinal, metabolic, genital, urinary, and other hormone systems, and your brain - are all affected by changes in your estrogen levels. And because your body is a delicate fabric of interlaced systems, each affects the other through a complex pattern of feedback loops that monitor and control your biochemical processes. Your body always knows when something is off balance, and it will send you messages to let you know it knows.

When your hormones are off balance, the first and most noticeable signs of that imbalance are, surprisingly enough, quite often not physical, but emotional changes. You feel off, not quite "yourself", but you're not exactly sure why.

After treating thousands of women for more than 35 years, I understand now that those emotional changes are often either a precursor to, or an accompaniment of, physical changes caused by fluctuating hormones or, as in the case of menopause, the result of dwindling hormones. So no matter what your friends, husband, or even your doctor may tell you, I am here to tell you right now, that what you are feeling is true and real, and it's absolutely not in your head.

You are feeling off because your hormones are off.

Chapter 3

The Estrogen Debate

Facts do not cease to exist because they are ignored.

Aldous Huxley

ESTROGEN AND BREAST CANCER

I'll wager that like just about every woman who comes to see me for the first time with menopausal symptoms, you're wondering if estrogen replacement will give you breast cancer, because that's what you heard on the news, or from a friend, or your mother, or even from your doctor. Well the answer is no. In fact, recent research shows that short term estrogen may actually protect women from breast cancer. I'll explain how, and why the benefits of estrogen have been so widely misrepresented and misunderstood in a bit. But first I want you to understand why I believe so strongly in estrogen replacement therapy. Here are some facts.

A drop or decline in blood estrogen levels, such as the one that occurs after child birth, (postpartum), and during peri-menopause and post-menopause, may lead to early symptoms of estrogen deficiency including physical, psychological/emotional and cognitive symptoms (something I call the "Estrogen Withdrawal Syndrome"). Women report hot flashes, night sweats, sleep disturbances; they experience anxiety, moodiness and/or depression. Cognitively they may note poor concentration, short term memory loss, and some find they can't think clearly. They feel "off," and their metabolism slows dramatically. That slower metabolism is why so many women become frustrated with the extra 15 to 50 pounds many tend to gain during the menopause; a slower metabolism means the weight is harder to lose.

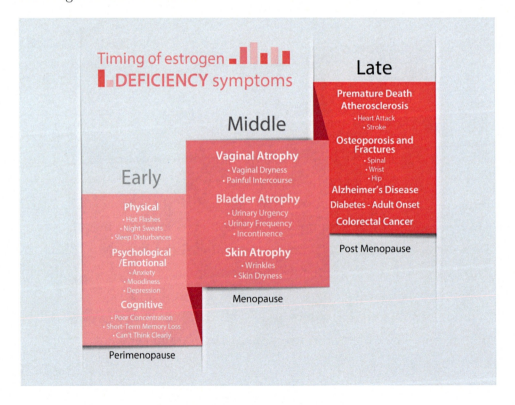

Estrogen Withdrawal Syndrome is also responsible for changes in bones, skin, heart and brain. We know, for example, that when post-menopausal women are chronically deprived of the estrogen hormone, their bones become more brittle, their vagina and skin become thinner and wrinkled, and their heart and brain arteries build up plaque. This lack of estrogen increases their risk of premature death, atherosclerosis, and subsequent heart attack and stroke, osteoporosis and fractures, Alzheimer's disease, adult onset diabetes, and colorectal cancer.

But an incredible thing happens when estrogen is replaced. It's almost like jumping into a personalized Fountain of Youth. Dry, wrinkled skin fills with collagen, plumps, and looks dewier, younger, and healthier.

Restoring estrogen quite simply means restoring and improving your quality of life, and the research now shows estrogen even extends your life expectancy.

So why in the world is there so much controversy about estrogen and hormone replacement therapy, and where did all that scary information about breast cancer come from?

A SHORT HISTORY OF ESTROGEN

Estrogen therapy first attracted controversy during the 1960s, when birth control pills were popularized. Greater sexual freedom for young women came at an unexpected price. The high-dose synthetic-estrogen and progestin birth control pills, combined with their "Madmen" type lifestyle of cigarettes and cocktails, were killing them. The deaths of those young women meant doctors learned by trial and error that too much oral estrogen and progestin can cause problems that lead to stroke, heart disease, and blood clots in the circulation. That's why today's birth control pills contain just a fraction, only 20-33%, of those earlier, and potentially deadly high doses.

So estrogen's first "black eye" came in the sixties when high dose birth control pills proved dangerous, but medical research showed much smaller doses of estrogen could be just as effective at preventing unwanted pregnancy. Then a second estrogen-related issue was publicized in 1975, when two articles in the New England Journal of Medicine reported that the use of Premarin (the estrogen created from pregnant mare's urine) after menopause was associated with an increased risk of well-differentiated endometrial cancer of the uterus. These articles led to a 50 percent decrease of estrogen prescriptions in the following five years, and close to 15 million women stopped their estrogen treatments between 1975 and 1980. Then researchers discovered that combining estrogen with a synthetic progestin (Provera), or preferably the biologically identical progesterone, eliminated the risk of cancer of the uterus, and estrogen replacement therapy again became a safe option for menopausal women.

In my own practice, I've only used the natural biologically identical hormones estradiol and progesterone since 1982. These natural vegetable sources still make up only a small portion of the post-menopausal hormones used in America today, even though, as you'll learn shortly, synthetic progestins like Provera may increase your risk of breast cancer.

HARVARD NURSES HEALTH STUDY

To find out more about estrogen and progestin's long-term affects on life after menopause, Dr. Frank Speizer of Harvard launched the Nurses Health Study in 1976, enrolling more than 121,000 thirty- to fifty-five-year-old nurses and following their hormonal regimens for twenty years. Twenty years later, at the start of the follow-up study in 1996, 70,000-plus menopausal women still remained in the study group. And we now know that these women who started taking estrogen or estrogen plus cyclic progestin at the usual time (within five years of menopause), for the usual reason (to reverse their menopausal symptoms), live longer and have healthier hearts than women who never used hormones. They experienced a 50% reduced risk for heart attack, and a 37% reduced risk for mortality.

Most women experience Menopause, (their last period), when they're about 51 years old. The Nurses' Health Study showed anyone who delayed starting her estrogen or estrogen plus progestin therapy more than ten years after menopause had less protection against heart attack. So we learned that women who began their hormone replacement therapy before or at menopause lived longer, and lived better lives.

And what about the women who had never used hormones before? How did they compare to the women who used hormones? Well, their risk of heart attack was low until age 54, but between the ages of 55 and 59, the risk of heart attack had increased by 50 percent, and by age 60 to 64, by 100 percent. The risk continued to increase as these post-menopausal women who never took estrogen aged.

What does that tell us? That when it comes to protecting your heart, estrogen or estrogen plus progestin therapy should be started during peri-menopause or within five years of menopause. More importantly, it tells us that estrogen or estrogen plus progesterone therapy means living a longer, healthier life.

ESTROGEN, MONKEYS, MENOPAUSE AND HEART DISEASE

In the 1980s, Dr. Tom Clarkson and colleagues wanted to find out how adding estrogen affected the hearts of menopausal women, because earlier human studies had shown that estrogen appeared to protect women against heart attacks. Since monkeys are close to humans in their genetic make-up and female monkeys also have a 28 day cycle, Dr. Clarkson investigated what happened to monkeys' heart arteries after their ovaries had been removed. These well-designed studies created a surgically induced menopause in the monkeys, who had been fed a typical American diet, one that is high in fats.

There were two groups of surgically-induced menopausal monkeys. One was given estrogen in the form of Premarin, a single dose that mimicked the same single dose most symptomatic, menopausal women take in pill form. The other group of monkeys served as the control group, and did not receive estrogen. That way Dr. Clarkson could compare data from the two groups and note any differences. And there were definitely differences - differences that supported the findings of the Harvard Nurses Health Studies.

Dr. Clarkson concluded that when Premarin was initiated within two years of a surgical menopause in the monkeys, estrogen reduced the plaque buildup in the heart arteries by 70%. Plaque buildup results in a disease known as atherosclerosis, or hardening of the arteries, which can then lead to heart attack. That's 70 percent reduced plaque build up in the coronary arteries with estrogen! However, if estrogen was delayed more than two years after menopause in the monkeys, the protection against plaque buildup was significantly reduced. Two years in a monkey is equivalent to five to six years in a human. That's a very important thing to note.

Dr. Clarkson's work dovetails nicely with the Harvard Nurses Study, because both the Nurses Health Study and the monkey data confirmed that if estrogen was to protect against plaque build up (atherosclerosis) and subsequent heart attack in women, it had to be started before menopause or early after menopause, ideally within five years. Dr. Clarkson was the first to describe this "window of opportunity" to initiate estrogen or estrogen plus progestin therapy in order to prevent plaque build up and subsequent heart attack.

I tell you this, because by 1990, more than thirty separate human observational studies conducted over the course of twenty years had shown that women who chose to take estrogen or estrogen plus progestin therapy at the usual time, within five years of menopause, for the usual reasons, to relieve their menopausal symptoms, had a 30 to 50 percent reduced risk of heart attack when compared to post-menopausal women who had taken no hormones.

The use of Premarin for estrogen therapy was not only found to eliminate the early menopausal symptoms but also subsequently reduced the risk for heart attack, premature death, osteoporosis, Alzheimer's disease, and colorectal cancer with long term use. Post-menopausal estrogen use appeared to increase both the quality of life and longevity. And even though Premarin was documented to increase the risk for blood clots and gallstones, these risks were rare when it was initiated in young, healthy, symptomatic women before or within five years of menopause.

So dozens of studies over decades show that estrogen replacement therapy means a longer, healthier life, especially when it comes to heart health. But estrogen is not the only hormone that can help you live your best life.

Just wait until you hear about the benefits of testosterone.

Chapter 4

Testosterone:

The Sexy Secret

Zest is the secret of all beauty. There is no beauty that is attractive without zest.

Christian Dior

TESTOSTERONE

Although the name testosterone wasn't coined until 1935, its powerful effect on the male of the species has been recognized for hundreds and perhaps even thousands of years. Aside from its influence on the maturation of the male sex organs (specifically the penis and scrotum), testosterone is also responsible for the physical development of facial and body hair, the deepening of the voice, for muscle mass and strength, and less obviously, for increased bone density. In addition, testosterone has long been thought to make men generally more aggressive than women. So my female patients are surprised that, not only do women also naturally produce testosterone in their bodies (in the ovary, adrenal gland, and elsewhere), but that in the vast majority of cases I will recommend that they add testosterone to their hormone replacement therapy regimen to significantly enhance their quality of life.

I think of testosterone as the sexy, secret icing on the estrogen hormone replacement cake. Testosterone can increase your energy, your motivation, your zest for life, your sexual interest (your libido), and your sexual pleasure.

I am happy, energized, and excited about life. My husband and I have the best sexual relationship ever. Bravo for the estrogen patch and testosterone replacement therapy! I wish that I had known about individualized bio-identical hormone replacement therapy five years ago.

Maggie

WHAT YOU DON'T KNOW ABOUT TESTOSTERONE

I originally discovered the power of testosterone in 1982, when I conducted a small study of 25 women under the age of 40, all of whom had a hysterectomy and both ovaries removed, resulting in them having a surgically induced premature menopause. These young menopausal women were the ideal group to study, because I wanted to know for certain whether the symptoms I saw in my peri-menopausal patients, who were for the most part in their forties or early fifties, were due to hormonal changes or were simply an adjunct to the aging process.

I am a very curious person, and I consider myself to be a life-long learner. That's probably what attracted me not only to medicine, but to the research side of medicine. In fact, my medical career began in academic or research medicine at the University of California San Diego Medical Center. For years, it was my job and my pleasure to ask questions, and then find answers about how our bodies work. I am always eager to learn all I can, so when 25 relatively young women, all of whom had undergone a hysterectomy and removal of both ovaries before age 40, creating a surgically induced menopause, arrived at my private practice within a month or two with the complaints of the same symptoms, I, true to my nature, was curious. I wanted to learn what they were experiencing and why.

I started by asking questions, all based on how they felt before and after their ovaries and uterus were removed. Prior to their surgeries, each of these young, healthy, vibrant women told me she enjoyed a 10-out-of-10 hormonal quality of life. However, shortly after their surgically induced menopause, none of them enjoyed a 10-out-of-10 quality of life; indeed, the quality of their life had plummeted dramatically.

Without estrogen, these women reported scores that ran from 0-3 out of 10.

Women taking some form of Premarin reported scores of from 4-6.

Two women in the group of 25 were taking pure estradiol shots (estradiol is the most prevalent form of estrogen naturally occurring in the non-pregnant female body throughout the reproductive years), and they both scored 7.

So no estrogen was very bad. Using oral Premarin gave them some relief, and shots of bio-identical estrogen replacement scored slightly higher.

Still, 23 of 25 women in my small study reported that their quality of life was 6 or lower, out of a possible top score of 10 (the quality of life they enjoyed before their surgeries). This didn't make sense to me. I could understand that the women who were receiving no estrogen at all would have a variety of issues and problems that would lead to a low quality of life, but what was baffling to me was that the women who were receiving various doses of estrogen in the form of Premarin weren't exactly enjoying the quality of their life either.

I decided to spend more time with each of these women in my study, reviewing their records, examining them, running tests, asking questions, and above all listening to what they were teaching me. I quickly realized that these women all shared the same basic set of complaints. They told me that they had no reserve energy, that they were exhausted by late afternoon or early evening. Their libido, or their interest in sex, was nonexistent, they suffered from reduced motivation, and they had lost their zest for life. Without prompting from me, each of my patients told me that they were not themselves. In addition, my physical examinations revealed that the skin of these women was dry, and their hair had lost its natural oil.

As I reviewed the lab results for my group of patients, I realized that the one bio-chemical that was undetectable in all 25 women was their serum testosterone level. They had no measurable, naturally occurring testosterone in their bloodstreams. Women normally produce testosterone in their bodies, although it is usually at levels much less than those observed in men, and it plays an important role in their overall well being, but I didn't know at the time how important.

TESTOSTERONE PIONEER

I searched the medical literature for any information I could find about the medical use of testosterone in women, and I discovered that a former professor of endocrinology at the Medical College of Georgia, Dr. Robert Greenblatt, had pioneered this field of study and practice in the 1940s. Other studies conducted after Dr. Greenblatt's groundbreaking work all pointed to one conclusion: testosterone is the hormone that has the greatest impact on the level of human sexual desire or libido, both in men and in women.

Dr. Greenblatt told me of a gynecologist located in Palm Desert, California, who was also using bio-identical testosterone and estradiol pellets for his wife and other women in his practice. These pellets were implanted under the skin in the fat tissue, which is a technique developed and used by Dr. Greenblatt for 40 years. When these small pellets of bio-identical estradiol and testosterone, each about the size of a grain of rice, are implanted into the fatty tissue under the surface of the skin, they dissolve very slowly, over a period of three to six months, providing a steady release of estradiol and testosterone into the circulation.

MY OWN RESEARCH

I obtained a supply of the estradiol and testosterone pellets and asked the patients in my informal study if they would be interested in seeing if we could restore the quality of their life by inserting bio-identical estrogen and testosterone pellets under their skin. They all readily agreed and signed consent forms. Once I had the informed consent, I implanted two estradiol 25 mg pellets and one testosterone 75 mg pellet under the skin of all these young women. After administering a local anesthetic, I made a small, 1/4-inch incision, inserted the hormone pellets, and applied an adhesive Steri-Strip to close the wound and covered it with two band-aids in the form of a cross.

Within a week after I implanted the hormone pellets in my study group, I heard back from my patients. All of the women reported that their quality of life was back to normal or 10 out of 10! They said they felt like themselves again. This was the first time I had ever administered testosterone to women, and it was encouraging for me to know that their quality of life had been brought back to what they said was normal.

It's interesting to note that many women experience low testosterone symptoms and low testosterone blood levels at an average age of 42; that is five to ten years before menopause.

Over the years, I have seen that a woman's zest for life and her libido or interest in sex can be directly tied to her testosterone levels. I have found improving libido often requires higher testosterone levels, while improving the overall quality of life and just feeling "good" can be achieved with somewhat lower doses of testosterone.

Beyond the benefits of increased energy, zest for life, and increased libido, I have discovered over the years that when a woman's early menopausal low-estrogen symptoms are about 90 percent resolved, introducing testosterone into the hormonal replacement mix can actually improve her low estrogen symptoms from 90 to 100 percent. So testosterone is perhaps even more important in hormone replacement therapy than most physicians and their patients realize.

ONE MORE THING

Testosterone also has a huge, hidden, virtually unknown benefit for women. Very few doctors realize that testosterone can actually increase a woman's bone density, can strengthen her bones, and is the most powerful tool we have to prevent osteoporosis and fractures in post-menopausal women. I have given testosterone pellets to many women over the last 30-plus years, and they have the strongest bones of any woman their age. Many are now above the 97th percentile for bone mineral density for women their age. When you think about it for a moment, this makes perfect sense. Men naturally have stronger and denser bones than women, and men have much higher testosterone levels than women.

After my hysterectomy not only did I have hot flashes all the time, but I also experienced anxiety, mood swings, depression, poor memory, and a feeling of not being well. My hormones were totally depleted and my life was falling apart. Four months of trying to help myself failed. The estradiol patch controlled my hot flashes right away. The testosterone shots I received also helped with many of my other symptoms, and soon I had my life back. It was like a miracle! I feel younger and healthier. Thank you so much!

Jo Ann

ANDROPAUSE

As testosterone began to improve my female patients' quality of lives, giving them back their motivation, their energy, (and especially when it perked up their libido and began to bring their sexy back) these happy women started bringing their husbands and partners back to my office. They believed that what's good for the goose is also good for the gander. So in 1982, I expanded my previously woman's only practice to include bio-identical hormone replacement therapy not just for the female menopause, but also for the so called male "menopause": andropause.

One of the problems I have discovered in trying to discuss andropause with men is that most men usually are not as aware of their mind, body, and spirit as women. Women have had to be very aware of their bodies because of their menses and the symptoms associated with hormonal changes that related to their menstrual cycle. Men don't have this same level of awareness of their own bodies. In fact, I've noticed that men traditionally tend to be less proactive than women in seeking wellness and more reactive, often only showing up in a physician's office because of a serious medical crisis. As a result, the first men I treated for andropause were husbands or partners of my female patients, but that has expanded over the years to include both married and single men who have heard about the benefits of testosterone replacement therapy, and once having experienced those benefits, have chosen to continue it as a regular part of their lives.

I find that many men with low testosterone levels feel angry and frustrated and that these symptoms often subside with physiologic doses of bio-identical testosterone replacement. Perhaps these men know that there is something inherently different, but they don't know what it is and as a result, they feel frustrated. Once the testosterone is replaced, their frustration defuses and they too feel more like their "original self."

NATURAL "VIAGRA"?

The decline in testosterone with andropause is usually the trigger for decrease in the frequency or firmness of a male's early morning erection. Many aging men have impotence, a problem maintaining an erection, and it's this impotence that has so quickly made Viagra a household name. I believe Testosterone replacement in men actually has many more benefits than Viagra. Testosterone offers physical, sexual, psychological, and cognitive improvements to middle-aged men with low testosterone after they start on testosterone replacement. Benefits include increased energy, increased muscle tone, and increased endurance for exercise. That enables men to lift heavier weights, increases muscle mass, and burns fat to increase the body's muscle-to-fat ratio. Testosterone also increases a man's libido, restores his early morning erections, and gives men more frequent and harder erections. Testosterone often also enhances their sense of well being, with less anxiety, depression, and moodiness, and allows men to sleep deeper and feel more rested when they awaken. It also increases their motivation and many men on testosterone replacement report they think more clearly, are better able to stay focused and complete tasks, and their short term memory improves as well.

Men's Awareness Calendar

Daily Symptom Rating Scale

Name _____

Age _____

Month/Year _____

Empty box = No problem	
1 1= Mild — Does not interfere with normal activities	
2 2 = Moderate — Interferes with normal activities	
3 3= Severe — Unable to perform normal activities	

Calendar Date		1	2	3	4	5	6	7	8	9	10	11	12	13	14	15	16	17	18	19	20	21	22	23	24	25	26	27	28	29	30	31
Low Testosterone	Decreased energy																															
	Decreased muscle tone																															
	Decreased endurance																															
	Decreased libido																															
	Reduced frequency AM erections																															
	Decreased firmness AM erections																															
	Sleep disturbances																															
	Headache																															
	Palpitations																															
	Increased body fat																															
	Decreased motivation																															
	Anxiety/Irritability																															
	Nervousness/Tension																															
	Crying/Hypersensitivity																															
	Mood swings																															
	Depression																															
	Problems coping																															
	Poor concentration																															
	Difficulty completing tasks																															
	Short-term memory loss																															
	Forgetfulness																															
	Can't think clearly																															
High Testosterone	Overly aggressive																															
	Road rage																															
	Violent																															
	Outburst of anger																															
	Red faced																															
Other Symptoms (add your own)																																
Stress	Psychological stress																															
	Exercise																															

Testosterone Dosage	1	2	3	4	5	6	7	8	9	10	11	12	13	14	15	16	17	18	19	20	21	22	23	24	25	26	27	28	29	30	31

Healthcare Provider's Recommendations: _____

CASE STUDY IN MALE CASTRATION

The first male I put on the testosterone implants was a young, thirty-three year old who was born with an undescended testicle. The testicle had been surgically removed when he was an an infant because of the high chance it would later become cancerous. When he was in his early 30s, this patient slid into third base playing baseball and tore his remaining testicle so badly that it, too, had to be surgically removed. He was, and is, the only male I have ever met who had known normal testosterone levels, but who was then forced to experience life as a male with neither testicles nor testosterone.

I learned from him that castrated men without testosterone can have hot flashes, night sweats, anxiety, irritability, moodiness, depression, declines in cognition, decreased energy, decreased libido, and decreased muscle tone. Sound familiar? These are all the same symptoms my female patients reported with a decrease in estrogen and testosterone following their surgically-induced menopause. That's why I believe the reactions to surgical castration in men is very similar to the reactions of surgical castration (the removal of ovaries) in women. The only difference I observed is that testosterone seemed to provide the benefits in men that both estrogen and testosterone alone produced in women.

While there are some contra-indications for the use of testosterone replacement therapy in men, the majority of men have no problems. I, of course, do complete workup of my male patients to screen for potential pre-existing issues that would preclude treatment with testosterone. Some of those issues include elevated blood count, liver disease, an existing prostate cancer, or high risk for heart disease. But I have found the mental, sexual, physical, and spiritual changes for men who receive testosterone replacement can be quite profound, life-changing, and long-lasting, both for the men themselves, and for their partners.

Testosterone replacement has been for me, a true eye-opener. It has led to a physical, as well as a spiritual awakening. It is amazing the clarity of thought, endurance, memory, love, and the ability to realize what was lost and now is found. I have new vision that allows me to see through the mental fog.

Charles

Chapter 5

One Size

Does Not Fit All

Somebody once said we never know what is enough until we know what's more than enough.

Billie Holiday

THE ESTROGEN WITHDRAWAL CONTINUUM

When your body begins to go into menopause, or into what doctors call the peri-menopausal state, it naturally slows down your body's production of estrogen, and that is a trigger for Estrogen Withdrawal Syndrome. Coincidently, every month during your pre-menstrual state, as part of your body's orchestration in preparation for a possible pregnancy in the days before your period begins, you may also experience Estrogen Withdrawal Syndrome in the form of PMS.

I believe that PMS, peri-menopause, menopause, and post-menopause are all part of a continuum, and all are triggered by estrogen withdrawal, resulting in physical, mental, emotional and cognitive issues.

I am also very aware that since we are all individuals, hormonal fluctuations in your body can also be affected by your environment, and by the way you live your life. Your weight, the kinds of food you eat, your exercise habits, alcohol consumption, drugs, and cigarette use, as well as the psychological factors in your life, like stress at work, relationships with your children, husband or significant other, your friendships, and even your attitude towards life itself can all contribute to erratic hormone levels, and intensify the symptoms of Estrogen Withdrawal Syndrome. Changes in exercise, nutrition, and simply reducing everyday stress can help tremendously, and can help to bring balance to your life. And everyone is different, so the amount of hormone you need replaced, or your dose, may be different for you than your sister or friends.

That's a critical piece of information you need to have, because one size does not fit all when it comes to hormone replacement therapy.

It never has.

BEWARE OF ORAL HORMONES

Of course, many thousands of doctors today already routinely prescribe hormones to their female patients. But remember, what most of these doctors are prescribing is something quite different from what I recommend and I myself prescribe to my own patients. These doctors are prescribing synthetic oral hormones, in specific, pre-determined doses of Premarin (estrogen) in pill form. I disagree with them. Here's why.

Doctors have known about the clotting problems with oral hormones since the 1960s. Remember that as young women started taking high-dose oral birth control pills, we saw a significant increase of heart attacks, blood clots, and strokes. When the original "estra-derm" estradiol transdermal patch became available in the 1980's, I switched all my patients who were on oral estrogens to the non-oral patch to eliminate the increased risk of blood clot formation.

French researchers have shown that transdermal estrogen eliminates the increased risk of blood clot formation in the circulation. This makes all the difference in the world when it comes to protecting women from needless harm, just by using a non-oral route of estrogen administration.

PILLS, PATCHES, CREAMS, AND GELS

Premarin, the estrogen made from pregnant mare's urine, comes in a pill form, in various doses. Premarin .625 mg is the most widely prescribed form of estrogen in the world.

There are two reasons why I never prescribe oral Premarin, unless a patient comes to me already taking it, and preferring it.

First, I've found that hormones administered in pill form aren't nearly as effective as the non-oral estradiol patch, cream, or gel which is absorbed instead through the skin. Here's why. When you take an estrogen pill, it is first filtered through the digestive system, broken down in the stomach, and then transported via the portal blood circulation to the liver, where it is screened, and up to 90 percent of the estrogen is immediately metabolized or broken down by the liver and excreted.

So only about 10 percent of the actual oral estrogen dose gets released into your general blood circulation to be distributed throughout your body. This is a very inefficient system, and it's also dangerous. When your liver is exposed to the full 100 percent dose of estrogen, it triggers the release of clotting factors formed in your liver into your general blood circulation. Those clotting factors can and do create blood clots in your general blood circulation. If the blood clots travel to your heart arteries, you could have a heart attack. If they travel to the brain, then that could lead to a stroke. And if clots travel to the lungs, pulmonary embolism, which is a life threatening situation, can result. That's exactly what happened in the early 1960's; that's why the young women on high doses of birth control pills died. Their livers were exposed to dangerously high levels of estrogen, which triggered the release of clotting factors that caused them to die prematurely of heart attack, stroke, and pulmonary embolism.

But when you use a transdermal gel, patch, or cream, the hormone is absorbed through the skin directly into the general blood circulation. It means you only need a fraction of the estrogen dose to be effective and safe. Why? Well remember, the liver's filtering process means only about 10% of the estrogen in pill form actually gets released into your blood circulation. So you can eliminate the over-exaggerated amount of estrogen exposure to the liver that occurs with oral estrogen, and instead give much smaller trans-dermal doses.

The second reason I never prescribe Premarin is I don't like the way the pregnant horses are treated in order to collect their urine, especially when we have bio-identical hormones readily available from natural vegetable sources. While it's true that Premarin is indeed processed in the laboratory from a substance produced by a living animal (the urine of a pregnant mare), Premarin also contains many other forms of estrogen and its metabolites that are good for pregnant horses, but are not naturally found in non-pregnant menopausal humans.

I use a different approach, one that combines bio-identical hormones, (which are the same as the hormones found in human females in every way) with a safer and a more efficient transdermal delivery system.

BIO-IDENTICAL HORMONES

When it comes to hormone therapy, I believe the best hormones are those that are natural, and from plant sources. It just makes sense because they also have the exact same chemical structure as those hormones produced by a woman's body, meaning that they are biologically identical, or bio-identical.

I prefer using a transdermal method of delivery, by means of a patch, cream or gel, because it means you can take the lowest dose possible to start your hormone replacement. What's more, it's easier to adjust a transdermal dosage than it is to adjust a pill, and that's something I think is absolutely critical. Just as one dosage amount of the hormone insulin is not appropriate for every diabetic every single day, one dosage amount of the hormone estrogen is not appropriate for every peri-menopausal or post-menopausal woman, every single day.

THE BENEFITS OF A COMPOUNDING PHARMACY

Bio-identical hormones prescriptions are generally filled at a compounding pharmacy. Compounding pharmacies are a lot like old fashioned pharmacies, and as such can formulate specialized cream or gel products with custom-made individualized concentrations of each hormone for each unique woman. The hormone cream or gel is dispensed with either a transdermal one-cc syringe system for gels, or a Topi-Click dispenser for creams. The Topi-Click applicator is about the size of and resembles a roll-on deodorant. Each of these methods allows you to adjust your individualized dose of each hormone and you can fine tune the dosage daily depending on your specific needs. This is what every diabetic does with insulin. She fine tunes and adjusts the dose to her specific needs every day.

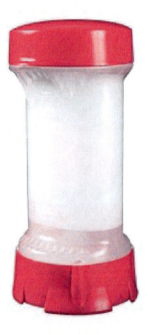

I always recommend each woman starts with a very low concentration of a hormone, and then gradually applies more product every three to five days, until her exact ideal dose is obtained. Once the individualized exact ideal dose is found, the compounding pharmacist can adjust the increased amount of hormone in the cream or gel so less product can be applied each day to produce the same, life changing results.

My aim is to concentrate the creams so that you take just one click per day. There are 120 clicks in each chamber of "topi-click". That means a four month supply of your estrogen, testosterone or progesterone each would cost you approximately $30. That is less than $100 per year for each hormone and I believe it to be one of the best $100 you'll ever spend on yourself, because it will help you to feel like yourself again.

DO THE TWIST

Many women enjoy the convenience of topi-click because it's so easy to use. Remove the cap and dispense the hormone cream by twisting the clicker at the bottom of the container, then apply the cream to your skin surface like you would a stick deodorant. A word of caution to women who are extremely sensitive and require an "exact amount" of hormone each day: the gel is more accurate in precise dosing and it is usually even less expensive.

This type of customized formulation from a compounding pharmacy often means you'll pay much less than insurance co-pays for your hormones, but remember, these compounded prescriptions are individualized to your own specific needs, which I believe is a key plus. I also think it's also important to note that there are licensed compounding pharmacies all over the United States and throughout the world, so this is an option readily available to anyone.

I have worked extensively with pharmacist Joe Gartner at the Good Pharma Compounding Pharmacy in San Diego to formulate these hormonal concentrations, all of which make it easier for you to apply and are more economical and safer than oral prescriptions. Once you have been stabilized on each individualized product, the hormones can often be combined together into one cream or gel for convenience. Joe has been dispensing bio-identical hormones for more than 30 years.

THE IMPORTANCE OF INDIVIDUALIZED DOSES

The original assumption that a fixed dosage of single Premarin pill would work for all women is both naïve and foolish. It is more appropriate for each woman to be treated according to her precise needs, rather than traditional medicine's fixed formula of one-size-fits-all dosage. In addition, I believe it's absolutely imperative to have the ability to fine tune your ovarian hormone replacement by independently adjusting your own dose daily if necessary.

Think about it this way. Every woman knows that one size does not fit all when it comes to bras. The female form comes in all shapes and sizes; you wouldn't give a woman with a breast size of 36DD a bra in a 32A size. It simply wouldn't support her properly. It's the exact same thing with hormone replacement. All women are different, and have different hormonal needs. In fact, in my patients I see a 300-fold spectrum of difference in doses between women who need the least to the greatest amount of estrogen for their replacement therapy. In other words, one woman may take a single dose, and another may need 300 times that amount. Not 300 percent more; that would mean only triple the dose. I do mean 300 times more. That's why individualized doses are so important.

Unfortunately, if you are at either of these extremes, and require either much lower or much higher doses than Western medicine's norms, you may have difficulty finding a healthcare professional to work with you. Why? Because you are "outside the box."

What's more, there are some days—particularly stressful holidays, and family or work pressures or even an increase in exercise—that will trigger a temporary need for a slightly greater dose of estrogen or testosterone. In the same way a diabetic "knows" when she needs to adjust her dose of insulin, I trust my patients to know when they need a bit more, and I trust them to fine tune their dosage daily if necessary, according to their specific needs. All I am doing is trusting my female patients in just the same way doctors would trust a diabetic to individualize her insulin hormone dosage to meet her changing and specific needs every single day. I believe it's absolutely critical that hormone doses be individualized in order for you to live your best life, because there are some days you will absolutely need more hormones than others. I prescribe two separate clickers of estrogen for most of my patients. One is to use daily, but I tell them that the second clicker, which is a weaker concentration of estrogen than their daily clicker, is simply to help them on "off days". The daily clicker contains more concentrated estrogen, and the second "boost" clicker, a weaker concentration which they can use to fine tune their dose on days of added stresses.

For me, hormone replacement was started immediately after my hysterectomy. I did not worry about taking estrogen because my doctor educated me thoroughly about the benefits, as well as the risks and side effects of the various forms of hormone replacement available to me. My estradiol patch delivers the estrogen directly into my bloodstream and bypasses the liver. The estradiol patch has "evened me out" emotionally. The edge has gone and there does not seem to be any underlying anxiety. I am physically comfortable and have been on the patches for 13 years. My estradiol dosage has been reduced gradually over the years and my estradiol levels are monitored each year with a simple blood test. My advice to you is to "be gentle with yourself."

Susan

Chapter 6

The Estrogen Connection

I am not afraid of storms for I am learning how to sail my ship.

Louisa May Alcott

YOUR LIFE AFFECTS YOUR HORMONES

As a researcher at the University of California, San Diego, my team wanted to study how the impact of fluctuating hormone levels affected a woman's quality of life during PMS. So out of a group of dozens of women with significant PMS symptoms we found and recruited the six women who had the most severe PMS symptoms we could find. We also recruited six women who had no history or symptoms of PMS at all. These symptom-free women were to be our control group. Our intention was to compare the hormone levels of the women with severe PMS with the control group, to see exactly what triggered the PMS.

Each woman agreed to a seven-day hospital stay, which was timed so that they would all have their periods on about day five of the hospitalization. We monitored each woman via blood samples every two hours for the entire length of their seven-day stay. They were admitted to the Clinical Research Center unit at the University Hospital. They weren't sick, so they were able to order whatever food they wanted, their beds were made for them, they were allowed to walk outside; in short, these women were on vacation from their normal lives. They were relaxed, and away from their day-to-day routine. And guess what? The six women with a previous history of severe PMS, the women who were specifically chosen because they suffered the most severe PMS symptoms of all the women we had interviewed, all had basically a PMS-free cycle that month.

What we found after examining all of those blood samples was that both groups of women all had basically the same hormone levels. There was absolutely no difference between the women who previously experienced severe PMS and the women who had no PMS.

So what happened? Why did the women who normally experienced severe PMS have a PMS-free cycle? As researchers, we thought we'd experienced our worst nightmare, there was no difference, we had no differentiating hormone levels to compare. But in reality, we were given tremendous information; we just didn't understand it at the time. We had taken women during what they said was routinely the most stressful time of the month for them, and we pampered them.

Why did that make such a difference? At the time I was confused, but in retrospect, this gives me insight about the power of environment and stress on hormones. The women in our study were stress-free, outside of their usual pressures of family, work, and everyday situations. Their hormones didn't react, and that meant they were free of their PMS symptoms. And because we thought we had failed as researchers to show hormonal differences, we never published this data. That was a mistake. We didn't find what we were looking for, so we failed to see and report what we were shown. This was a new truth revealing itself and now I see it clearly. The absence of stress for these women also meant an absence of their PMS symptoms. Stress impacts hormones. Your life impacts your hormones.

PMS AND MENOPAUSE: THE SAME, BUT DIFFERENT

It's important to remember that the human body is an incredible, complex life force with an amazing ability to self-adjust. Our research showed us that by changing your diet or environment, or by adding exercise, by breathing fresh air and taking in Vitamin D from the sun, you can help to alleviate or reduce PMS symptoms.

Menopause is different than PMS because your body isn't ebbing and flowing with hormones; it has actually lost ovarian hormones because your ovaries simply aren't making as much of them. But the body does have that innate ability to self-adjust, and it can adjust to menopause. So you have a choice. As a menopausal woman you could simply wait for your body to balance itself, but, as your mother or grandmother can tell you, that can take years, or even decades. What's more, you could likely experience mid and late low estrogen symptoms and medical conditions and those symptoms include vaginal dryness, painful intercourse, urinary urgency, loss of urine, thinning skin, and wrinkles. There are other potential dangers. Medical conditions resulting from long term low estrogen include premature death, atherosclerosis (or hardening of the arteries which can lead to heart attack or stroke), osteoporosis and fractures, Alzheimer's Disease, adult onset Diabetes, and colorectal cancer.

So the real question to ask yourself is whether you can or should wait out the hormonal storm and suffer through what may turn out to be months or even many years of physical and emotional effects; or if you can and should bring balance back to your body by giving it what it no longer produces enough of on its own.

The only way to "cure" Estrogen Withdrawal Syndrome is to replenish it with exactly the one thing that it needs - estrogen - to gently supplement your body with natural hormones as its own production decreases.

CHANGING HORMONES MEAN CHANGING METABOLISMS

The biggest problem I see menopausal women experiencing is the tremendous weight gain many have, often 15 to even 50 pounds in the year or two around menopause. The weight gain is definitely fat in the abdominal and thigh regions and fat is a source of estrogen. I believe this extra fat women seem to put on during menopause may be because their bodies are trying to maintain a healthy level of estrogen. As their ovaries wind down estrogen production, the body may make up for it by increasing its fat production. If this is the case, I believe that by augmenting with bio-identical estrogen and keeping those estrogen levels consistent, your body won't need to manufacture estrogen from your fat. That means we may be able to eliminate some of that weight gain that accompanies menopause.

Remember, the weight gain at menopause has been shown in part to be due to a decrease in a woman's metabolism. That's why I believe the war against menopausal weight gain is best fought with an increase in exercise, with focus on the abdominal and thigh muscles. Dieting does not increase a woman's metabolism; exercise does. If you're experiencing this kind of weight gain, I encourage you (and all Peri-menopausal and menopausal women) to do sit ups, abdominal crunches, Pilates, Yoga, and Pelvic Tilts to prevent or reduce the abdominal obesity, and to do exercises similar to the Thigh Master to burn fat off your thighs.

Please, take control of your own destiny. Always keep your hormone levels close to their pre-menopausal levels, and do it naturally. This is an important contributing factor to being able to take charge of other aspects of your life. Menopause is a great time of freedom!

Reese

Chapter 7

The Women's Awareness Calendar

We have only today. Let us begin.

Mother Teresa

HORMONES AND GOLDILOCKS

I consider the Women's Awareness Calendar to be the single most important tool I have used over the decades to help women balance their hormones. It's a daily, weekly, and monthly record of symptoms, each of which is correlated to a specific hormone. The calendar works on the Goldilocks principle, because remember, I individualize doses, and we're trying to find the hormonal zone for you that's "just right." The calendar tells us immediately if you have "too little" of a specific hormone, or if you have "too much," and that helps us determine what we need to do in order to adjust your dosage so that you're hormonally "just right." We want to eliminate post-menopausal symptoms of too little hormone without side effects of too much hormone.

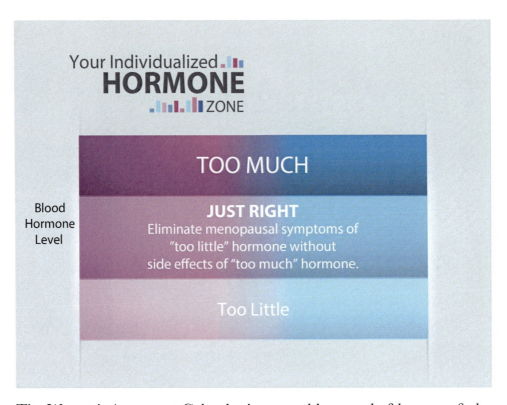

The Women's Awareness Calendar is a monthly record of how you feel on a daily basis, and you can start it on any day of the month. Use it, and you'll begin to see patterns of symptoms, so it's really, really important that you're deliberate and consistent about filling it out every day! If something significant occurs in your life - for example you lose a loved one, your job, or your marriage; you move, or if your in-laws move in, if your children go off to college or come home to live - make an asterisk on that date on the top of the calendar and write a quick note on the back of the Women's Awareness Calendar and detail what happened. Why? I have found that your emotional health affects your hormonal health and visa versa, so you may find you'll need to adjust your hormones to ease these life stresses. Knowing what triggers the stressors, and knowing that you can adjust your hormones to help you with those stressors, is important information for you and your doctor to have.

Your careful monitoring of the daily changes in your symptoms will help you to determine the right amount of each hormone you need to achieve your individual hormone zone.

UNDERSTANDING YOUR BODY

The Women's Awareness Calendar is for all women to use no matter where they are in their reproductive lives and I hope you will share it. It's a wonderful gift for a mother to give her daughter, allowing her to learn about, and understand what is happening with her body as it changes from a girl into a young woman. Many of my patients are ending their reproductive cycles as their daughters begin theirs. Seeing the physical, mental, emotional and cognitive issues that pop up around their daughter's periods and their own menopause can be critical information for both mother and daughter, because they often show a pattern of symptoms. These patterns help us to know when the hormonal danger zone is coming, whether it's from PMS, or Peri-menopausal symptoms, and that knowledge is powerful. It means you can anticipate those rockier times of the month and you can prepare for them as you cycle. Post-menopausal women have no cycle, so every day is basically the same, they have low, or possibly no hormones.

QUIGLEY
FOUNDATION

Women's Awareness Calendar

Daily Symptom Rating Scale

Name_____

Age_____

Month/Year_____

		1	2	3
	Empty box = No problem	**1= Mild** Does not interfere with normal activities	**2 = Moderate** Interferes with normal activities	**3= Severe** Unable to perform normal activities

Calendar Date		1 2 3 4 5 6 7 8 9 10 11 12 13 14 15 16 17 18 19 20 21 22 23 24 25 26 27 28 29 30 31
Low Estrogen	Hot flashes	
	Night sweats	
	Sleep disturbances	
	Headache	
	Palpitations	
	Vaginal dryness	
	Frequent/Urgent urination	
	Anxiety/Irritability	
	Nervousness/Tension	
	Outburst of anger	
	Crying/Hypersensitivity	
	Mood swings	
	Depression	
	Poor self-esteem	
	Fear of losing control	
	Problems coping	
	Poor concentration	
	Difficulty completing tasks	
	Short-term memory loss	
	Forgetfulness	
	Can't think clearly	
High Estrogen +/- Progesterone	Breast fullness	
	Breast tenderness	
	Feeling bloated	
	Nausea	
Low Testosterone	Decreased energy	
	Decreased libido	
	Decreased vitality	
	Decreased motivation	
	Dry skin	
High Testosterone	Acne	
	Increased facial hair	
	Lowered voice	
	Loss of scalp hair	
Other Symptoms (add your own)	Weight gain	
	Joint aches and pains	
Stress	Psychological stress	
	Physical activity (exercise)	
Menstruation	Mark X at onset of period	

Hormone	Individualized Dosage	1 2 3 4 5 6 7 8 9 10 11 12 13 14 15 16 17 18 19 20 21 22 23 24 25 26 27 28 29 30 31
Estrogen		
Progesterone		
Testosterone		

Healthcare Provider's Recommendations: _____

_____

_____

_____

HOW TO USE THE WOMEN'S AWARENESS CALENDAR

The Women's Awareness Calendar enables you, like Goldilocks, to find Your Perfect Hormonal Zone for each hormone. That's the hormone range where you are symptom-free and feel great without any side effects. The more you make the calendar your own, the more quickly you'll become aware of your symptoms, their patterns, and which treatment helps you or gives you specific side effects. Remember, every woman is different, and the key to successful hormone replacement therapy is individualized doses, knowing your body and what it needs. So learn which symptom(s) you experience when there is "too much" or "too little" of each hormone. For example, "too much" estrogen can cause you to feel breast fullness and/or tenderness, while "too little" can cause hot flashes, moodiness, and/or a loss of cognition.

Many times, even though you feel one symptom is the primary difficulty you are having, you may have to use a second or third related symptom as a more reliable guide to determine whether your hormone level is actually "too high" or "too low" because "too much" or "too little" of the same hormone may cause the same symptom. A good example for that is headaches. Too much estrogen or too little estrogen can both be a trigger for headaches, so those secondary and tertiary symptoms will help you to determine whether today's headache is from too much or too little estrogen.

Make sure you identify the severity of each of your symptoms on the calendar: 1 for mild, 2 for moderate, and 3 for severe symptoms. Leave the individual square empty if you are not affected by that symptom that day. Eventually we are aiming to have a blank calendar. You are then in each of your individual hormonal zones.

Towards the bottom of the calendar, where it indicates "miscellaneous," add any symptoms you experience that aren't already listed there. Next, record your daily stress level, psychological and physical activity (exercise). Again, use a simple scale of 1,2,3: 1 indicates mild, 2 moderate and 3 severe stress. Below these recorded stress levels, mark X at the onset of your period if you are still having cycles and below that, in a separate box, write in any hormones, prescription drugs, or homeopathic remedies that you are taking to see if they are helping or hindering your progress.

YOUR PERSONAL HORMONAL ZONE

As you become familiar with your body's response to each hormone, you will start to notice that the subtlest indicators may represent the best clues to your needs. You must be patient when first establishing your Hormonal Zone. Start with one hormone at a time, and keep daily records of your progress on the Women's Awareness Calendar. The Calendar can help you to tune into your own body and validate how you're feeling, but only you can really know how each hormone works best for you, and whether it is too little or too much today.

For women who are still menstruating, it takes at least one full menstrual cycle to see the benefits or side effects of estrogen therapy, and three to four months to fine tune the various hormone replacement amounts, delivery methods, and timing of the hormone dosage with respect to the time of the cycle.

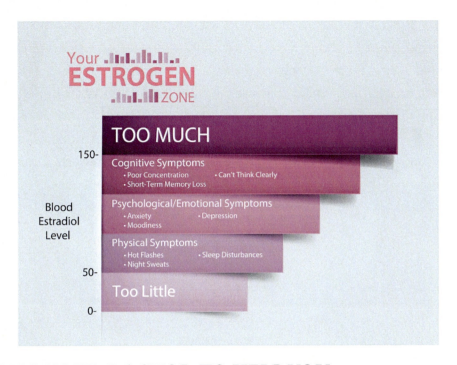

HELP YOUR DOCTOR TO HELP YOU

If you choose hormone therapy, you may need to help educate your doctor or healthcare provider about the value of the Women's Awareness Calendar, so follow these guidelines:

LOWEST DOSE. Have your healthcare provider start you on the lowest effective dose of each natural, bio- identical hormone, initiated one hormone at a time.

ESTROGEN FIRST. Start with estrogen first. The right dose will reverse many of your physical symptoms almost immediately. Your psychological, and emotional symptoms may take a bit more estrogen, and the cognitive issues often take even a bit more estrogen. The goal is to find your individual zone, the one that improves all your symptoms, the physical as well as the emotional and cognitive issues you're facing.

We are looking for the lowest dose of estrogen that eliminates your low-estrogen symptoms 95 percent of the time, taking into consideration the normal everyday stresses you experience. The other 5 percent of the time I consider to be major life stresses, such as the holidays, children leaving home, changing jobs, a death, or divorce. During these stressful times, it's natural for you to need a little extra dose of hormone, which I give you permission and the freedom to administer by yourself. Establishing the right estrogen dose will help improve your self-confidence and your self-esteem.

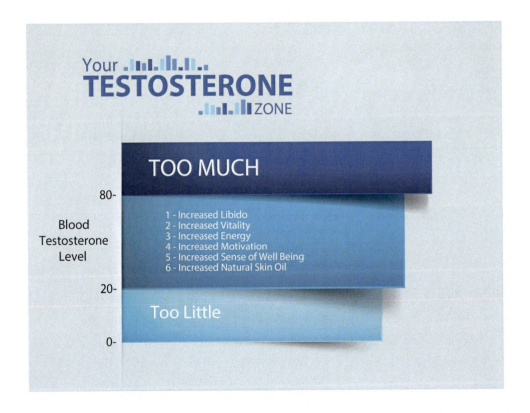

TESTOSTERONE NEXT. Add testosterone second. This will increase your libido, vitality, energy, metabolism and your sense of well-being. Testosterone will also restore natural skin oil production. Estrogen alone can give you a sense of well-being, but the testosterone is the sexy secret icing on the estrogen hormonal cake, and provides the vitality, your zest for life, your joie de vivre. I typically give both estrogen and testosterone in the morning to improve your daytime symptoms.

PROGESTERONE LAST. Progesterone is added last to post-menopausal women who still have their uterus, with the understanding that it may result in renewed menstrual bleeding and possibly PMS symptoms. I also give the annual menstrual calendar to all pre-menopausal women and to post-menopausal women taking progesterone, because they still have their uterus.

Record any bleeding you have every day of the calendar year and distinguish it between light flow (O), normal flow (X), heavy bleeding (solid square), or spotting (S). Take progesterone at night, before bed, because it often helps you get to sleep. All post-menopausal women with their uterus intact need to take some form of progesterone if they take the normal estrogen doses. I tend to prescribe one to two clicks of progesterone (50 mgs per click) at bedtime to post-menopausal women with their uterus intact if they take the normal estrogen doses. I don't typically start PMS or Peri-menopausal women on progesterone if their cycles are regular and normal or light in flow. They are still producing adequate progesterone from their ovaries. However, once their periods get heavy or space out more than six to eight weeks apart, I will add progesterone at bedtime.

It is important to be aware of the options available in the timing and methods of application of various forms of estrogen or estrogen plus progesterone therapy. Most of your PMS/peri-menopausal-menopausal/post-menopausal symptoms will improve or cease within a few hours or days of that particular blood hormone level reaching your specific Hormonal Zone, but if you suffer from vaginal dryness and bladder urgency and/or stress incontinence, know that you'll need a little patience. These symptoms take two to six weeks to reverse, because the estrogen needs time to stimulate increased tissue growth in those areas.

Menstrual Record Chart

Name _____ Year _____

	Amount of Flow: X Normal	O Light	■ Heavy	S Spotting	No. of days from start of period to beginning of next

Month	1	2	3	4	5	6	7	8	9	10	11	12	13	14	15	16	17	18	19	20	21	22	23	24	25	26	27	28	29	30	31	
Jan.																																
Feb.																																
Mar.																																
Apr.																																
May																																
June																																
July																																
Aug.																																
Sep.																																
Oct.																																
Nov.																																
Dec.																																

Dr. _____

KEEP TRACK AND ADJUST YOUR DOSE

Tracking the daily amount, time, and method of administration of estrogen or estrogen plus progesterone therapy allows you and your healthcare provider to know the most effective timing for administering each hormone. You will be able to tell how long it takes for that hormone to enter and leave your blood stream.

The beauty of estrogen or estrogen plus progesterone therapy is that when we use natural hormones to replace or replenish levels that are faltering or absent, we can do a blood measurement to determine whether the natural hormone you are taking is actually getting into your bloodstream in the amount you need to feel and be your best. Blood levels themselves do not necessarily have a perfect correlation with the hormonal effect, but if you do decide to test your estradiol blood level, know that it should be above 50 pg/ml for estrogen to prevent osteoporosis and heart disease.

NOT ALL TESTS ARE EQUAL

A word of caution: in the last few years, a saliva test has been described as "better" than blood hormone testing in assessing a woman's hormonal status. I have had patients record their symptoms via the Women's Awareness Calendar and then I have had both blood and saliva testing done simultaneously. To date, I have found a much closer correlation between the calendar record of their symptoms and their blood hormone levels than from the saliva tests. In fact, there have been times when the saliva tests indicated the hormone measurement was too high, while the blood test and symptom records indicated the hormone was too low, and vice versa. But even blood levels can be deceiving, because they can only tell you what is occurring at that moment in time.

Getting a blood or saliva test is like taking a single snapshot of your hormonal health, whereas the Women's Awareness Calendar gives us a much bigger picture of what's going on with your body. It's much more like a movie, and that means we can more easily see your body's reaction to the amount of hormones you've replaced, so we can help you adjust your dose accordingly.

JUST RIGHT!

Think of it this way. When you're trying to determine your perfect dose of bio-identical hormones, it's like you're in a shower with only one handle to adjust the hot and cold water. You start out with cold water adjusting the temperature up gradually. Find out if it's still too cold or if you've overdone it with the hot water and you need to adjust it back a bit, and make it a little cooler. Too little hormone is like the cold water in the shower; to make it just right, you have to add more hormone. If you add too much hormone, just like the hot water in the shower, you dial it down, making adjustments until you've found a hormonal amount or temperature that is comfortable. That's exactly what we're doing by adjusting your individualized dose of each bio-identical hormone to meet your specific needs.

The ultimate goal is to find your perfect individual dose, or your perfect hormonal zone for each hormone.

This is one of the key differences between traditional hormone replacement therapy and the method I use. I individualize. In fact, I empower my patients to eventually regulate themselves, and to adjust their daily dosage much in the same way a diabetic checks, adjusts, and fine-tunes her insulin. Initially a diabetic needs a doctor's help in determining when and how much insulin to take. However, she eventually learns better than her doctor exactly what works for her because she knows her own body. Estrogen and testosterone replacement are similar. Eventually you will know what you need better than your doctor, just like a diabetic does. But first you need to use the

Women's Awareness Calendar to know what indicates "too little" or "too much" of each hormone for you. Get to know your body. Learn to maintain each of your hormonal zones. It's a common-sense approach that has tremendous benefits and positive results.

INDIVIDUALIZED DOSES FOR L.I.F.E.

As a physician, one of the very first questions I will ask you when you come for a consultation is whether or not you are regularly menstruating. Your monthly flow can tell me a lot about your health. Your period, or your lack thereof, can be a signal that you are approaching menopause, or that there is something wrong—especially in women who are under the age of 51. Skipped periods or erratic bleeding can be your body's indicator of several things. It may show us whether your ovarian age is older than your chronological age; meaning you're approaching menopause, or it can tell us that you're stressed out, too thin, or less likely, perhaps even seriously ill.

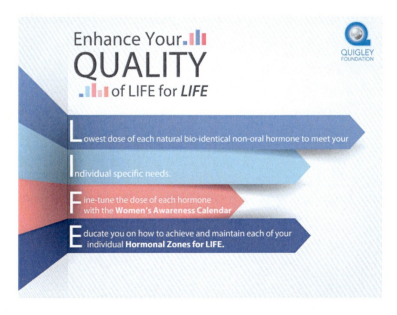

These are all factors that we must take into account when determining whether or not you are a candidate for hormone replacement therapy, and if so, what dosage is right for you.

My goal is to find the exact dosage that is right for you — the amount of hormone that will get you into and keep you in your zone. I recommend individualized Hormone Therapy for LIFE:

Lowest dose of each natural biologically identical non-oral hormone to meet your

Individual specific needs.

Fine-tune the dose of each hormone with the Women's Awareness Calendar.

Educate you on how to achieve and maintain each of your individual **Hormonal Zones for LIFE.**

Always, we want to give you the lowest dose of estrogen, tailored to your individual needs, that will eliminate:

(a)   physical signs and symptoms,

(b)   psychological and emotional symptoms, and

(c)   cognitive symptoms.

I know from my decades of experience that it usually takes less estrogen to eliminate the physical symptoms than it does to eliminate the emotional and cognitive issues. So when I hear researchers say estrogen therapy has no effect on emotional or cognitive issues, I know it's because the researchers are prescribing too low a dose of estrogen to reverse those emotional or cognitive symptoms or issues.

My aim is to reverse all of your physical, mental, emotional and cognitive symptoms to achieve your perfect Estrogen Zone.

KNOW YOUR BODY

Your body is constantly creating a delicate balance with regard to the hormones that ebb and flow throughout your system, and that's especially true when it comes to the relationship of hormones to stress. That's because stress increases your heart rate, which increases the blood flow throughout your body. Remember: hormones are produced by one organ, and they enter the bloodstream to travel to every cell throughout your body. So as the heart rate increases, the blood flow also speeds up. As a result, your kidneys work faster filtering your blood, and greater concentrations of your hormones are excreted in your urine. Any increase in your heart rate may reduce the blood hormone levels in your body.

Even something as seemingly random as a fever or extra duration or intensity of exercise can also increase your heart rate and lead to decreased hormone levels. That's why diabetics need extra insulin when they increase their exercise and why they may also need more insulin when they are experiencing additional stresses in their lives. And that's why I give women on hormone replacement therapy the same respect, courtesy, and trust as most physicians today give to diabetics. I allow them to adjust their doses to ensure that they are always in their perfect hormone zone, something that's easy for them to track with the Women's Awareness Calendar.

MINDFUL OBSERVATION

After they've been on hormone replacement therapy for a month or two, and after they're feeling like themselves again, I want to make sure my patients are aware of what it feels like to be even slightly estrogen deprived. I know that their estrogen levels will inevitably change, whether it's the result of holiday stress or even just a little extra time at the gym. The important thing is to be aware of what it feels like when those changes occur and estrogen levels are falling.

So I ask my patients to take what I call a day of "mindful observation" on a stress-free day, a weekend or a day off work, to become aware of the slight changes that can be early warnings of more significant issues. To begin this exercise, I ask my patients to remove their patch or delay their estrogen cream or gel for a few hours. I then ask them to keep track of how they're feeling by chronicling any changes every hour or two with their Women's Awareness Calendar. In most cases, it doesn't take long for these patients to feel "different." This experience gives them a solid understanding of those first symptoms that tell them they're off, and it gives them a baseline to help them to make adjustments early as needed to stay within their perfect individualized Hormonal Zone. I invite you to go through the same mindful observation process, so you, too, can ensure that you will always maintain your perfect individualized hormonal zone.

I began using natural, biologically identical hormone replacement to treat migraine headaches that coincided with my monthly menstrual cycles. I was in my early forties at the time. The hormone therapy brought the immediate relief that no migraine medicine could—and I had tried everything! I am now approaching my tenth year of hormone therapy and I am still peri-menopausal. I love having the ability to self-adjust my estrogen dose by trimming or adding a small portion of patch, as needed. It makes perfect sense to allow my dosage to fluctuate along with my body's natural changes.

Peggy

Chapter 8

Women's Health Initiative, Estrogen & Breast Cancer: The Truth

A lie can travel half way around the world while the truth is putting on its shoes.

Mark Twain

A SHOCKING ANNOUNCEMENT

The Women's Health Initiative was launched in 1991 by the National Institutes of Health, and was the largest, most ambitious, and most expensive study of its kind ever, with an initial budget of close to 725 million taxpayer dollars, and a final bill that is expected to reach a billion dollars or even more. It was an attempt to comprehensively test the effects of Hormone Therapy, Diet Modification, and Calcium/Vitamin D supplements on post-menopausal women's health.

That's why I was stunned when on July 9, 2002, I learned that the National Institutes of Health had abruptly and prematurely stopped one of its four groundbreaking Hormone studies, the Prempro Clinical Trial. It was big news that made even bigger international headlines, because according to the press release and the media frenzy that followed, it was stopped because "Women on the estrogen plus progestin therapy had a 26 percent higher incidence of breast cancer," "a 41 percent increase in strokes," a "29 percent increase in heart attacks," and a "doubling of rates of venous-thromboembolism" (blood clots in the circulation). In addition, the head of the Women's Health Initiative study said "the increased risk applied to all women, irrespective of age, ethnicity (or) prior disease status".

I was especially rocked by this last, blanket statement. So were millions of shocked and terrified women, who panicked and stopped taking their hormones cold turkey immediately. In fact, it's estimated that more than half of all the post-menopausal women world-wide stopped their estrogen replacement within a year of that ominous announcement. And those shockwaves continued to ripple, reaching beyond women who were currently using hormone replacement therapy, because it also meant that millions of other younger, symptomatic menopausal women never started any type of hormone replacement therapy at all because they, or their doctors, were afraid of the possibility of breast cancer, heart attack, stroke or blood clots in the circulation.

This announcement changed menopausal management world-wide.

My experience with my patients and my practice had shown me that when women begin their individualized bio-identical hormone replacement therapy at about age 50, they lead longer, healthier, happier lives. That's why the date July 9, 2002 has been burned into my mind as a terrible day, second only to September 11, 2001. I feel the mishandling of the premature termination of the Women's Health Initiative Prempro study in 2002 was the greatest disservice western medical research has done to the menopausal women of the world. I know the consequences of July 9, 2002 have meant tremendous needless pain, suffering, and even the early death of tens of thousands, or perhaps even millions of post- menopausal women. And as you'll see shortly, I'm not the only physician who believes that.

ESTROGEN PROTECTS YOU

Because of the way the news was handled on July 9, 2002, you probably have the same fear as nearly every new, young, healthy, symptomatic peri-menopausal or early post-menopausal woman who has come to me since that day for relief from her menopausal symptoms. She is concerned that estrogen will cause breast cancer and premature death. Here's what I can now tell you. My own research, and all other research to date, indicates unequivocally that for young, healthy, symptomatic women who begin their hormone replacement therapy before or within five years of menopause, estrogen therapy is not only safe and effective at enhancing the quality of your life, it will likely increase your longevity too. Estrogen protects you.

Now a decade later, with the data of all four Women's Health Initiative Post-menopausal Hormone Studies available, there is one consistent, relatively unpublicized finding you need to know. When women began hormone replacement therapy before age 60, like 99% of my patients have done, all four Women's Health Initiative Post-menopausal Hormone Studies show they had a consistent 30% decreased death rate from all causes of death compared to the placebo/control women. And those numbers apply whether the women are using estrogen alone or estrogen plus progestin. That means 30% fewer needless premature deaths with estrogen replacement. Estrogen therapy actually means a longer, healthier life. Those are the facts. This is what I have experienced working with menopausal women and estrogen therapy for four decades.

So why did the Women's Health Initiative get it so wrong?

I think it was a perfect storm of misunderstanding; on the part of researchers, the media, and the public. Unfortunately the findings were generalized to all post-menopausal women regardless of age. Researchers didn't segregate the participants with regard to age or symptoms, or health status, or even separate those older women in the study who were initiating their estrogen plus progestin therapy well past menopause - in some cases, decades past menopause. That's where the misunderstanding began.

AN UNUSUAL BACKGROUND

Although I am a Board Certified Reproductive Endocrinologist, and a Board Certified OB/ GYN, I began my professional career as a Clinical Researcher. That's unusual; most doctors choose either to see patients, or to conduct research and rarely move from one discipline to the other. I have had the opportunity to do both.

As I've mentioned earlier, I've always been a curious person, and that curiosity has served me as a physician, because when I moved from academic research into private practice, I continued some of my research habits. The Women's Awareness Calendar is a perfect example of this melding of medical research into medical practice. I have, quite literally out of habit, gathered data from thousands of completed calendars from thousands of women. Each of these calendars shows my patients' symptoms before and after they begin their hormone replacement therapy, and tells me how much hormone each and every woman needs to take to eliminate her physical, psychological, emotional and cognitive issues. They give me information about the range of hormone doses I have found to be effective, and as I have told you, I see a 300-fold difference between the woman whose symptoms are eliminated with the least amount of estrogen, to the woman who needs the most amount of estrogen.

The data from these Women's Awareness Calendars is an incredible resource. I've learned, and continue to learn, so much about women and how their hormones affect them because of that data. That's why I was so shocked by the findings of the Women's Health Initiative's Prempro Clinical Trial. I knew from my own decades of research and data that transdermal, individualized, bio-identical hormone replacement therapy was, quite literally, a lifesaver for many of my patients.

Bottom line? I guess I'll always be kind of a nerd when it comes to research. I always want to know what happens if? So I not only read all the new studies in my field of expertise, I actually am one of only a very few doctors I know of who has an obsession to dig between the lines and carefully examine the numbers in a research paper to uncover important golden nuggets of information that are relevant to my patients. And that's what I decided to do with the data from the Women's Health Initiative Hormone Studies.

ONLY ONE VARIABLE AT A TIME

My research background gives me a deeper understanding of the way clinical research is conducted. Unlike most other physicians, I will always look at how a study was designed, who was studied, and the way it was implemented as I examine its results.

A primary rule of research is that you never introduce more than one variable at a time into any clinical study. Why? More than one variable means that it is impossible to see if there is a cause and effect relationship, and that's what clinical research is always trying to discover: whether "A" affects "B."

Think about it like this. Your toddler has a fever and you want to bring the fever down. So you give her a cup of herbal tea and an aspirin, and the fever goes down in 30 minutes. What returned her fever to normal? Was it the tea? Was it the aspirin? Or was her fever reduced because her body was recovering on its own? You can't know for certain, because you introduced two variables at once. Well, it's the same thing with clinical studies.

You can and should only test one variable at a time compared to a control or placebo group so you know and understand the relationship between the variable and the outcome. That's a critical piece of information to remember, as we examine what the Women's Health Initiative was, and what it was not.

First of all, it was only the Women's Health Initiative Prempro Clinical Trial which was terminated on July 2, 2002, which was just one of the four ongoing Women's Health Initiative Hormone studies. The other three studies continued. So the big question to ask is, why weren't the other studies stopped? Well, the answer is "Prempro."

WHAT IS PREMPRO?

Prempro is a single pill which combines two very different hormones: first, the estrogen Premarin, and second, the synthetic progestin, Provera. It gets its name from the combination of the two hormones Premarin and Provera, hence Prempro. You already know Premarin is an estrogen created from pregnant mare's urine. Well, Provera is a synthetic progestin, an anti-estrogen, meaning that the progestin opposes the action of estrogen on various tissues in a woman's body. For example, while estrogen stimulates growth of the tissue of the inner lining of the uterus, Provera blocks or inhibits that growth.

So in this one pill, Prempro, you have both an estrogen, and an anti-estrogen, or two variables.

Do you see the problem in giving both an estrogen and an anti estrogen in the same pill? What you are studying can either be affected by the estrogen Premarin, or by the anti estrogen Provera. It's impossible to differentiate, and furthermore, in the case of Prempro, the two variables may actually oppose each other. That's a huge red flag to me as a researcher; it makes me question whether the results of the Prempro study were caused by estrogen (Premarin) or the synthetic progestin, the anti-estrogen (Provera). As with the toddler's herbal tea and aspirin, you simply can't know what was responsible for your results.

But since researchers were looking at the effects of hormones on menopausal women, that meant some of those women needed to take the second female hormone, progestin. Recall that earlier studies had shown that menopausal women who have a uterus and are taking estrogen only have an increased risk of a specific type of uterine cancer. Giving them a progestin, or an anti-estrogen, substantially reduced that risk. So when the Women's Health Initiative set up its groundbreaking clinical hormone studies, it separated women into two groups: those women with a uterus who took estrogen plus progestin and women without a uterus who took estrogen only. I know this sounds like it's going to get a little complicated, since we're talking about four separate hormone studies, estrogens and anti-estrogens, but bear with me; the background information is really important.

THE "GOLD STANDARD" OF MEDICAL RESEARCH

In the Women's Health Initiative Hormone Clinical Trials, the women who still had their uterus received estrogen plus synthetic progestin in the single pill, Prempro, while women who had no uterus (those who had had a previous hysterectomy), received the exact same dose of estrogen in a Premarin .625 mg pill but no synthetic progestin or Provera 2.5 mg. Both groups of women, those taking Premarin and those taking Prempro, were observed and measured against a control group of women who received a placebo pill containing no hormones at all. This allowed researchers to conduct a "Double-Blind Placebo-Controlled Clinical Trial " which is considered to be the "Gold Standard" of Western Medical Research.

These kinds of clinical trials are extremely expensive and labor intensive. They cost many millions of dollars. Because of those huge costs, they generally last less than five years, and assess short term health risks and benefits. The Women's Health Initiative clinical trials, however, were slated to continue for eight years. Researchers choose eight years for the length of their study because they had done extensive statistics, based on the incidence of the various medical conditions they were studying, and they determined how many women of each age group (50's, 60's, 70's) they needed to gather enough data to reach a statistically significant difference between treatment and placebo groups. After all, this is the primary goal of all medical research, to study enough people long enough to have sufficient data to reach a statistically significant difference between the treatment and placebo groups.

Research data is statistically significant when the probability or "P-value" is equal to or less than 0.05. This means that the probability of the results happening due strictly to chance alone is less than 5 in 100. It's a number that's universally accepted amongst researchers, and one every researcher understands as being their goal.

CLINICAL TRIALS AND OBSERVATIONAL STUDIES

Short Term Clinical Trials in combination with Long Term Observational Studies are a good, reliable way to observe and measure the risks and benefits of a particular treatment. That's why both of the Women's Health Initiative Double-Blind, Placebo-Controlled Hormone Clinical Trials were also paired with the much larger, sister Women's Health Initiative Observational Studies. Now, these long term Observational Studies are very different than short term Clinical Trials. An Observational Study may last for decades and is based on observing what happens when people continue their usual self-determined behavior. In the case of the Women's Health Initiative Hormone Studies, the women were already either taking or not taking hormones, and the researchers simply observed and reported what they saw for the duration of the study.

You already know about one of the largest and longest running Observational Studies on women's health, the Harvard Nurses Health Study. Since 1976, nurse-participants have provided researchers with landmark data, giving them insights on how diet, exercise, and other lifestyle factors affect women's health. The study has followed women as they age, so the data includes a lot of good information about menopausal women and hormones, all of which was available to the researchers who designed the four Women's Health Initiative post-menopausal Hormone studies.

Now, you may have thought the Women's Health Initiative was studying women who are like you, and like my patients - the vast majority of whom are healthy and symptomatic between the ages of 40 and 55 when they approach me wondering "Is it safe for me to start hormones for my menopausal symptoms?" But you'd be wrong. Actually, only a very small fraction of the post-menopausal women studied in the Women's Health Initiative Prempro Clinical Trial was young, healthy, and symptomatic. And that, I believe, was another major problem with this study.

WHAT EXACTLY WAS THE WOMEN'S HEALTH INITIATIVE STUDYING?

Women's Health Initiative researchers were actually looking at a lot of different things that could affect women's health, including diet and vitamin supplements and there were many women who took part in more than one of the Women's Health Initiative Clinical Trials at the same time. In fact, 5,000 women participated in all three of the Clinical Trials at the same time, and 30% of the participants in the Women's Health Initiative Hormone Clinical Trials were also part of the Women's Health Initiative Diet Modification study. When it comes to research, one woman participating in more than one study at a time is a huge "no no." Why? Again, it's all about the variables. And in the Women's Health Initiative there were multiple variables.

If a woman changes her diet AND takes calcium and vitamin D supplements AND takes an estrogen AND an anti-estrogen, how can you possibly know the cause and effect of just one of those variables on her health? You can't, and as a researcher, I'm shocked that the post-menopausal women were allowed to participate in more than one clinical trial at a time. A major basic rule of clinical research is that a participant can only volunteer for ONE CLINICAL TRIAL AT A TIME. Still, I knew the Women's Health Initiative was an important milestone in women's health research. I was determined to find those gold nuggets of information the researcher in me knew were there.

In fact, after painstakingly examining the Prempro Clinical Trial data, I discovered that only about ten percent of the women studied were in any way relevant to my patients and to you. My experience in research told me that I would have eliminated 90% of the women chosen for this study because they were either too old, too unhealthy, asymptomatic or too many years post-menopause to initiate hormones and participate in these important clinical research trials.

THE WHO AFFECTS THE WHAT

I know from my years as a researcher that who we study can be as important as what we study, and that the "who" absolutely affects the outcome of the "what." Since the Women's Health Initiative Prempro Clinical Trial was studying the effects of the estrogen and synthetic progestin hormones on menopausal women, to me it only made sense to study women who were young, healthy and seeking relief from menopausal symptoms - that is those women who had the same basic characteristics as 99% of the women I see in my practice. The truth is, researchers who designed the Women's Health Initiative Premarin and Prempro Clinical Hormone Trials intentionally strongly discouraged women with moderate-to-severe menopausal symptoms from participating. Surprised? I was. So why didn't the researchers want to include symptomatic, menopausal women?

You should know that every woman who joined the Women's Health Initiative Premarin and Prempro Clinical Trials had a 50% chance of getting randomly assigned to the placebo or control group. These women would not be receiving any hormone at all for the entire proposed eight years of the study.

If you're a woman who is having significant menopausal symptoms such as hot flashes and night sweats, anxiety, irritability, moodiness, depression,or cognitive problems, would you be willing to risk giving up your current hormones, something you knew was working for you and providing you with symptomatic relief? Would you be willing to give up all of that relief for eight long years, knowing that you had a 50% chance of receiving a placebo? Probably not. The Women's Health Initiative researchers knew this, but they needed volunteers for their study, so they instead recruited much older, asymptomatic, unhealthy women who would be more likely to remain in the study. Then they had these older women initiate their single dose of Premarin or Prempro many years after their menopause, most of them for the first time in their lives.

WHAT DID WE REALLY LEARN?

When we look at the women who participated in the one study which was the cause of all the media hype, the Women's Health Initiative Prempro Clinical Trial, we find participants initiated their Prempro when they were from 50 to 79 years old, with an average age of 63. The average woman was 12 years post-menopause, and didn't have moderate to severe menopausal symptoms such as hot flashes when she first started her hormone therapy. In fact, only 12% of the Prempro participants had moderate to severe menopausal symptoms when they entered the Women's Health Initiative Prempro Clinical Trial.

The number of participants between ages 50-54 in the Prempro Clinical Trial was deliberately restricted to only about ten percent of the total women, even though this was the most clinically relevant sub-group. This was the data that I wanted to look at most closely. Why? The participants were the closest in age to the patients I see to initiate hormone therapy, but even they were very different than most of my patients, because only a small fraction of that ten percent actually had significant menopausal symptoms. Prempro participants did, however, have other issues. In contrast to the thousands of healthy women I have started on estrogen, the Prempro participants were very unhealthy.

* 36% had high blood pressure and were taking medication for it

* 20% were taking cholesterol-lowering medication

* 50% were previous or current smokers

* 34% were obese

* 4% were diabetics

* Incredibly, 7% had already suffered a previous heart attack

* Only 6% were current hormone users

* Only 20% had ever used hormones

Actually, only a very small fraction of a fraction of all of the women being studied in the Women's Health Initiative Prempro Clinical Trial mirrored my patients or any of the symptomatic women who classically take menopausal hormones.

All of the women in the Women's Health Initiative Prempro Clinical Trial got a single oral pill of Prempro with the exact same dose of both the synthetic estrogen Premarin .625mg, and the synthetic progestin Provera 2.5 mg. And remember, these two hormones actually oppose the action of the other. Premarin is an estrogen, and Provera is an anti-estrogen. You already know that I prescribe only individualized, non-oral bio-identical hormones and I don't believe in a one-size fits all dose; I individualize the dose of each hormone for each patient the same way we do for patients with other hormone deficiencies like diabetes. In fact, the diabetic analogy is appropriate, because I believe Western Medical Research would never allow a research study to be conducted to determine the risk/benefits of insulin in diabetics and

1.   Give sugar with insulin or diametrically opposing substances at the same time.

2.   Give one single dose of insulin to every diabetic. It would mean that the dose would be "too little" for some, "too much" for others.

3.   Delay and start the insulin an average of 12 years after the diagnosis of diabetes was made.

4.   Give insulin to humans who had no symptoms of diabetes or non diabetics.

But that's exactly what researchers did when they designed the Women's Health Initiative Premarin and Prempro Hormone Clinical Trials. They gave women Premarin, which is estrogen alone, or Prempro, which is estrogen with progestin, or an estrogen and an anti-estrogen, in a single dose, years or even decades after menopause, to women who had no menopausal symptoms.

CONTENT INTO CONTEXT

So, the study, for the most part, wasn't studying what it claimed to be studying. In fact, two of the leading researchers, Harvard's Joanne Manson, MD. and UCSD's Robert Langer, MD, both of whom were heads of Women's Health Initiative study centers, now say that the Women's Health Initiative Premarin and Prempro Clinical Trials were primarily designed to see if older women considerably past menopause would get the same benefits of hormone replacement therapy as younger women who started hormones within five years of menopause.

What's more, there were a number of variables that were being introduced into the study at the same time. As a researcher, not only was I deeply disturbed by the number of variables, I was also profoundly bothered by the fact that the participants were not representative of the vast majority of women who suffer from menopausal symptoms and consult their doctors about estrogen therapy. To me, that meant any conclusions needed to be carefully studied in order to put the content of the Prempro data into context.

It wasn't easy to do, especially based on the research findings which were presented on July 9, 2002 when we were told that "women on the estrogen plus progestin therapy had a 26 percent higher incidence of breast cancer" and "a 41 percent increase in strokes", a "29 percent increase in heart attacks" and a "doubling of the rates of venous thromboembolism" (blood clots in the circulation). Scary stuff, right? Well, not so much if you understand that research is first and foremost a numbers game.

These numbers, 26%, 41%, and 29% can be deceiving, because when I put on my researcher's hat and looked at the actual numbers behind those percent increases, and when I was able to put the content of the Women's Health Initiative Prempro data into context, I learned that story told on July 9, 2002 was deceptive. Very deceptive.

THE NUMBERS RACKET

The reality is, clinical researchers should only look at absolute numbers rather than express them as percentage, because the way the numbers are presented can make all the difference about how those numbers are perceived. When the absolute numbers in medical research data are small, researchers will often express their data as percentage differences to make their data appear more dramatic than it is. So let's break down those Prempro numbers, and let's start with what the researchers told us about the 26% increased risk of invasive breast cancer in Prempro users, because that's the number that scared and continues to scare so many women.

In the Women's Health Initiative Prempro Clinical Trial, when you look at the placebo or control group of non-hormone users, there were 30 breast cancers per 10,000 women per year. The placebo or control group shows us the baseline number of women with breast cancer that we would expect to see in the general population of all post-menopausal women aged 50-79 years who don't use hormones. The theory is that in any random group of 10,000 women, you would see about 30 of them with breast cancer. But in the treatment group, the group using Prempro, there were 38 breast cancers per 10,000 women per year, or an increase of 8 more breast cancers per 10,000 women per year compared to the placebo group. Here's where it gets tricky and here's where you'll be glad I have a research background.

That information of 8 additional breast cancers per 10,000 women can be expressed in several different ways. You can refer to it either as

8 per ten thousand women per year,

0.8 per thousand women per year,

0.08 per hundred women per year,

or as a 26% increased risk of breast cancer per 10,000 women per year.

To calculate the percent difference, we take the difference between the Placebo and Prempro groups, which is the number 8, and then divide that number 8 by the placebo group incidence of 30 and multiply that by 100 to express it as a percent. The result is a 26% increase in the Prempro group over the Placebo group (38-30=8: 8/30 X 100%=26%).

The truth is, the results of this study could have been reported by saying the women who used Prempro had an 8/100ths of one percent increased risk of breast cancer per year. Now, 8/100ths of one percent sounds very different than the 26% increased risk, but the numbers are both correct. Both are a means of expressing the same information. But the perception is that 26% portrays a greater risk than the minuscule sounding 8/100ths of one percent.

This is the numbers racket of medical research.

DATA AND SAFETY MONITORING BOARD

The Data Safety Monitoring Board did a terrific job of protecting the volunteers in the Women's Health Initiative Hormone Clincal Trials, and was responsible for pulling the plug on the Prempro Clinical Trial. It was an independent group whose job it was to review the data from the

Women's Health Initiative's Hormone Clinical Trials and to protect the participants from harm. Early on, it created a series of metrics, or artificial limits, with regard to what board members considered to be an unacceptable risk to the women in the studies. Every condition, heart attacks, colorectal cancer, breast cancer, even the death rate, had its own artificially created "line in the sand." The board decided that if either of the studies reached a limit for any of its risks, that study would be stopped immediately. And those limits were very conservative, because the board was determined to protect the participants.

Garnet Anderson, Phd, the bio-statistician who was in charge of the data from the Women's Health Initiative, said that "because breast cancer is so serious an event, (The Data Safety Monitoring Board) set the bar lower to monitor for it." When it came to breast cancer, Anderson said they were very concerned about making sure the women were safe. "We pre-specified that the change in cancer rates did not have to be that large to warrant stopping the trials. And the trial was stopped at the first clear indication of increased risk."

So the board set a very conservative level as it's "line in the sand" when it came to breast cancer and other health risks. It met every six months to review the data for both the Premarin and Prempro Clinical Trials, and to decide whether or not it was safe for each study to continue.

But remember, the "who" affects the "what," and "who" researchers were studying were, for the most part, much older, overweight, and even obese smokers who had previous heart disease issues and who had never used hormones before.

THE MEDIA AND THE RUSH TO PUBLISH

At its semiannual meeting on May 31, 2002, when the average volunteer was five years into the proposed eight year study, the Data and Safety Monitoring Board recommended that the Women's Health Initiative stop the Prempro Clinical trial because the breast cancer risk had crossed its pre- determined " line in the sand". Remember there were four hormone studies being conducted at the same time by the Women's Health Initiative, two Clinical Trials, the Premarin (estrogen only) and Prempro (estrogen plus synthetic progestin), and two sister Observational Studies, but only one of them was being recommended for termination.

Just six weeks after the Data and Safety Monitoring Board stopped the Prempro study, the Journal of the American Medical Association, or JAMA, published the findings of the Women's Health Initiative Prempro Clinical Trials on July 17, 2002.

This is highly unusual. Normally, a groundbreaking study like the Women's Health Initiative's Prempro Clinical Trial is vetted and examined carefully by peers of scientists, researchers and/or physicians in a thorough review process before publication. It usually takes time, a lot of time, to responsibly analyze, digest and carefully write such a pivotal, important study. But sufficient time and reflection, discussion and debate doesn't seem to have occurred following the termination of the Women's Health Initiative Prempro Clinical Trial. In fact, the article originally published in JAMA on July 17, 2002 was actually incomplete. It was missing the last ten weeks of Prempro data. Again, this is highly unusual, and I wonder why rush to publish.

I believe it was this rush to publish and the over-generalization and over-dramatization of the data, and the media publicity that followed, that caused the misinformation and misrepresentation of the actual facts.

So let's look at what the Women's Health Initiative Prempro Clinical Trial data really said about breast cancer. It appears now that the risk of invasive breast cancer begins after five years of use of Prempro. Prempro, which contains a synthetic progestin or anti-estrogen, increases the risk of breast cancer. Not estrogen. Not bio-identical progesterone. It was the synthetic progestin, **Provera**, which is in **Prempro,** that increased the risk of breast cancer!

SEPARATING FACT FROM FICTION

Now that all of the information is in and we can look at the data from all four Women's Health Initiative Hormone Studies, the Prempro Clinical Trial and its long term Observational Study counterpart of estrogen plus progestin, plus the Premarin Clinical Trial and its long term Observational Study counterpart of estrogen only, here's what the real truth is:

The Prempro Clinical Trial was stopped by the Data and Safety Monitoring Board early because it crossed its so-called "line in the sand" with regard to breast cancer danger. Normally when a study is stopped for medical reasons, the head researchers and the participants are immediately notified to stop any medication. That did not happen with the Prempro Clinical Trial. In fact, the 40 Women's Health Initiative Head Researchers didn't even know the study had been stopped for nearly a month; they were notified 28 days after its termination. Moreover, the vast majority of these head researchers had not examined the data or even read the paper until after it was already accepted for publication in JAMA. They seem to have been, inconceivably to me, actually excluded from the key research processes of analyzing the data, writing the paper, and putting the content of the Prempro data into context.

Even more disturbing to me is that the Prempro participants weren't told to stop their medication for 38 days. That means the Prempro participants continued to take their Prempro for more than a month after it was decided that it was too dangerous for them to continue in the study. What's more, participants received their notification letter to stop taking Prempro on July 8, 2002, the day before the July 9, 2002 Press Conference. The way the increased risk of breast cancer was hyped by the media created confusion and misunderstanding that continues today. Why? Because the news reports, especially television news reports, didn't give the whole story. They didn't differentiate estrogen only from estrogen plus the synthetic progestin, or Premarin from Prempro. Remember, the Data and Safety Monitoring Board did not stop the Premarin (estrogen only) Clinical Trial. It was allowed to continue, but because the media used the term "menopausal hormones" instead of identifying Prempro, women got the wrong message, and stopped taking their estrogen.

A DEADLY MISUNDERSTANDING

On October, 21, 2003, a little over a year after the initial publicity surrounding the Prempro Clinical Trial, Tara Parker-Pope of the Wall Street Journal wrote a piece entitled "The Case for Hormone Therapy." She said "in recent months, as additional data about the Women's Health Initiative study (Prempro) have emerged, critics have become increasingly vocal about what they see as flaws in the study. The strongest concern is that the women in the Women's Health Initiative were simply too old - and started hormone therapy too late in life - for researchers to come to any meaningful conclusion about the value of the treatment for women facing menopause" ... and that according to Elizabeth Lee Vliet, a Tuscon, Arizona physician and author of several books on menopause, "It's absolutely critical to point out that the Women's Health Initiative does not speak to younger women …You're looking at a 30-year age difference between the average menopausal woman who comes into my office versus [some of the] women that were in the Women's Health Initiative. It's like taking a group of old men at risk for prostate cancer and saying it applies to young men."

Parker-Pope continues her article with this positive note from one of the Women Health Initiatives researchers. "Nothing about this study should preclude women who need the hormones to take the hormones unless you're at very high risk," and, "Whatever was said 15 months ago, that's when it was a shock for everybody. We've had a year to calm down and get back to the fact that there still is a place for hormones for treating women." To put this into perspective, I have seen only a few women at "very high risk;" basically these are women who have already a breast cancer.

PROGESTIN AND BREAST CANCER RISK

Women's Health Initiative's Stanford Head Researcher, Marcia Stefanick, Phd. continued to look at the data from the Prempro and Premarin studies, and in a 2007 JAMA paper reported that when you compare the studies it "strongly suggests a role for progestin in relation to increasing breast cancer risk." Remember, Provera is a synthetic progestin, an anti-estrogen. In that same paper, Stefanick reported that women who took estrogen alone actually had a lower incidence of breast cancer. Again, it was Provera, not estrogen, that was linked to the increased breast cancer risk. Estrogen may actually protect against breast cancer, at least in the short term.

I think it's important to note that the synthetic progestin Provera is still to this day the most commonly prescribed form of progestin used world-wide. But remember, women with a uterus have a risk of developing uterine cancer when they take estrogen alone, so progestin, or Provera can be an important protection against that cancer. So, how do we determine the risk or benefit of estrogen plus progestin when it comes to breast cancer versus cancer of the uterus? My solution is quite simple. I use estrogen plus a natural, bio-identical progesterone, which I know is safer and protects a woman from cancer of the uterus.

How do I know this?

French researchers did a study in which they looked at women who were taking estrogen only, estrogen plus synthetic progestin, and estrogen plus a natural, bio-identical progesterone, and they compared that data to a control group of non-users. That study showed that the natural progesterone does not increase the risk of breast cancer, like the synthetic progestin does.

THE TRUTH ABOUT BREAST CANCER

In the short term (less than five years of use), neither Premarin (estrogen only) nor Prempro (estrogen plus synthetic progestin) increased the risk of breast cancer in post-menopausal women aged 50-79 years. However, when the synthetic progestin is added to estrogen the risk of breast cancer in the Women's Health Initiative Prempro Clinical Trial doubled with five to nine years of use, and tripled with more than ten years of use.

In the Women's Health Initiative's long term estrogen plus progestin Observational Study, when estrogen plus progestin was initiated in women at the usual time for the usual reasons, there were 40 more breast cancers per 10,000 women per year compared to the control group of non users (72 vs. 32 per 10,000 women per year). This increased risk with estrogen plus synthetic progestin is substantiated by both the British Million Women study and the French Teachers' Study which used other progestins.

In the British Study, there were 30 more breast cancers per 10,000 women per year than the control group of non users (60 vs. 30 breast cancers per 10,000 women per year). The French Study approached doubling the risk of breast cancer with the synthetic progestin compared to controls. In contrast, four major long term studies suggest estrogen has a much smaller risk to breast cancer than progestin.

The Harvard Nurses Health Study demonstrated that when researchers looked at estrogen use in five year increments, women who used estrogen only for less than 20 years we did not observe a statistically significant increased risk of breast cancer and that

1. The lower risk of breast cancer after 5-10 years of estrogen use was limited to heavier women

2. The increased risk of breast cancer with longer term use was greater in leaner women.

Heavier women, in this case, would be someone with a Body Mass Index, or BMI, that is greater than 30, and leaner women would have a BMI of less than 25. Average BMI, for the record, is anywhere from 25-30.

Both the Women's Health Initiative (long term estrogen only) Observational Study and the British Million Women study demonstrated a small increase of four more breast cancers per 10,000 women per year. This was much less than the 40 more and 30 more breast cancers shown in post-menopausal women with estrogen plus progestin in the respective studies. The French Teacher's study also reported that breast cancer risk was higher with estrogen plus progestin compared to estrogen only. However, the French were the only researchers who investigated the risk of estrogen plus natural bio-identical progesterone, and found it did not increase the risk of breast cancer.

BREAST CANCER RISK
per 10,000 women per year

	Estrogen Only	Estrogen Plus Progestin
SHORT TERM WHI Clinical Trials	**7 FEWER** benefit	**8 MORE** RISK
LONG TERM WHI Observational Studies	**4 MORE** minimal risk	**40 MORE SIGNIFICANT RISK**

PREMARIN: BREAST CANCER PROTECTION

After it terminated the Women's Health Initiative Prempro Clinical Trial, The Data and Safety Monitoring Board continued to conduct its assessments every six months to see if it was safe for the Premarin Clinical Trial participants to continue. It never did stop the Premarin study, but the study actually was terminated a year before it was scheduled to end by the National Institutes of Health. I feel the reason the Premarin Clinical Trial was stopped prematurely was because Premarin (estrogen alone) was very close to reaching a statistically significant decreased risk of breast cancer, not an increased risk. In fact, the research showed that estrogen only was 1/100th of a point from demonstrating a statistically significant decreased risk of breast cancer.

Remember when we talked earlier about the goal of all research to show a statistically significant difference between the control group and the treatment group? The number researchers are hoping to achieve is .05 (statistical significance). That's the magic number that takes us from chance to probability. And in the Women's Health Initiative Premarin Clinical Trial, it was the National Institutes of Health, NOT the Data and Safety Monitoring Board, that pulled the plug on the study when it reached a probability or P value of .06. That is only one hundredth of a point from demonstrating a statistically significant DECREASED risk of breast cancer with estrogen (Premarin) only.

MIXED MESSAGES

Why would the National Institutes of Health want to stop a study that was just about to show estrogen as a protection? I spoke to a member of the Data and Safety Monitoring Board and asked why this important information wasn't publicized with the same effort as Prempro. She said, "We didn't want to confuse the women."

We didn't want to confuse the women?

Remember, the Women's Health Initiative was the largest and most expensive Double-Blind Placebo-Controlled Clinical Trial ever done, and it had gotten a lot of press with the Prempro data. So if it had publicized its findings of estrogen as a protection against breast cancer, after implying it was a risk two years before in 2002, it would have meant reversing some pretty strong language. The head of the Women's Health Initiative and the National Heart Lung Blood Institutes, Dr. Jaques Rossouw, had already said that the adverse effects of Prempro, what the media referred to as "**menopausal hormones**", and its increased risks, including breast cancer, and heart attacks, applied to "… all women, irrespective of age, ethnicity, or previous disease status". But that statement was inaccurate at the time, nor is it accurate now.

NEUTRAL OBSERVATION

I believe the most critical component in research is that the researcher is a neutral observer. The data must be collected, examined, and shared and the integrity of the researcher must be above reproach. In the case of the Prempro and Premarin Clinical Trials, I do not believe the National Institutes of Health acted as a neutral observer. The way the data was released, and the misunderstanding of the data by the media, women and their doctors, combined with the fast track to publish, all combined to create the perfect storm of misunderstanding.

Archibald MacLeish says there is only one thing more painful than learning from experience, and that is not learning from experience.

What I have learned from my experience as a doctor and as a researcher is that it is absolutely critical to be a neutral observer. When we pollute a study with a hidden agenda, preconceived expectations, or by choosing specific participants to obtain a specific outcome, we are not neutral observers. I sincerely hope Western medicine is open to integrating the lessons taught by the misunderstanding, the rush to publish, and the media blitz of the Women's Health Initiative Prempro Clinical Trial so we do not make the same mistake of inflicting needless pain and suffering on menopausal women and their families ever again.

In a 2012 article, one of the Women Health Initiative head researchers, Garnet Anderson, PhD, published that in the Women's Health Initiative Premarin Clinical Trial, participants who took Premarin .625 mg (estrogen only) for an average of almost six years and then were followed for an additional six years for a total of 12 years, showed a statistically significant decreased risk of breast cancer and a statistically significant 63% decreased death rate from breast cancer, compared to women who took a placebo or no hormone at all.

Chapter 9

Estrogen: The Heart of the Matter

It is better to light a candle than to curse the darkness.

Eleanor Roosevelt

So now you understand the confusion and the truth about the Women's Health Initiative with respect to estrogen and breast cancer, but you probably have never heard that the primary purpose of both of the Women's Health Initiative Premarin and Prempro Clinical Trials was to determine whether estrogen or estrogen plus progestin protected women from heart disease, which is actually the number one killer of post-menopausal women. Five times as many women over the age of 60 will die from a heart attack than from breast cancer. You probably didn't know that, did you?

Women's Health Initiative researchers already were aware that more than 30 observational studies showed a 30-50% decreased risk of heart attacks in young, healthy, symptomatic, menopausal women who started taking their estrogen at the usual time (before or within five years post-menopause) for the usual reasons (to reverse menopausal symptoms). Both human and animal research data (remember the surgically-induced menopausal monkeys?) had suggested that there is a "window of opportunity" in which estrogen or estrogen plus progestin must be started to gain maximum protection to prevent heart attacks. So when the Women's Health Initiative Prempro Clinical Trial researchers reported that participants were experiencing a 29% increased risk of heart attack, rather than the protection most of us who were researching and actually prescribing these hormones expected to see, they did the same thing I did. They looked at both the "who" (the women who participated in the study) and they looked at the "what" (the numbers) and then they examined the data.

THE WINDOW OF OPPORTUNITY

The truth is that all of the current human and animal research, including the four Women's Health Initiative Hormone Studies, suggest that when women initiate their estrogen or estrogen plus progestin before or within five years of menopause, they reduce their risk of heart attack. However, if a woman delays the initiation of her estrogen or estrogen plus progestin well beyond that five year window of opportunity, she could actually increase her risk for subsequent heart attack.

Here's what we know. When a woman takes estrogen before or within five years of menopause, it delays the plaque build up in her heart arteries and prevents subsequent heart attack. Without replacing estrogen after menopause, the plaque tends to continue to grow and could eventually obstruct blood flow to the heart, or cause the plaque to dislodge. That's what causes blockages in the heart arteries and subsequent heart attacks. So the good news is if a woman takes estrogen early, before or within five years of menopause, she protects herself from plaque build up in her coronary arteries and subsequent heart attack.

The bad news, however, is if oral estrogen or estrogen plus progestin is started many years after menopause and the plaque has already begun to build up inside her heart arteries, this may then increase her risk of a heart attack during the first one to two years after the initiation of hormone use. That increased risk of heart attack may be linked to whether she experienced menopausal symptoms such as hot flashes. Women's Health Initiative researchers reported those at highest risk for heart attack are much older post-menopausal women who had been having moderate to severe hot flashes since menopause. These are women who had never taken estrogen or estrogen plus progestin, but were estrogen deficient for many years. If they then started their estrogen or estrogen plus progestin after age 70 or more than 20 years post-menopause, they were an **alarming 10 times as likely** to have a heart attack as an elderly post-menopausal women with no hot flashes. That is a **ONE THOUSAND PERCENT INCREASED RISK**. I tell you this because I want to emphasize that not all women need to take estrogen to prevent heart attacks. However, women experiencing moderate to severe hot flashes or other symptoms of estrogen deficiency may consider initiating estrogen or estrogen plus progestin at the usual time for the usual reason, within 5 years of menopause, to reverse their menopausal symptoms as a potential protection against plaque build up in their coronary arteries and subsequent heart attack.

THE WHO STILL AFFECTS THE WHAT

Here's the reality. Most women who are looking to start or who are currently taking hormones are much healthier and begin their therapy at a much younger age than the Women's Health Initiative Premarin and Prempro Clinical Trial participants.

My patients, who are representative of most women who are looking for relief from their peri-menopausal or menopausal symptoms, start estrogen therapy when their symptoms begin, on average when they're about 46 years old, or between the ages of 40 to 55 years. So my typical patient is pre-menopausal or within five years of menopause. In addition, she is experiencing moderate to severe menopausal symptoms. And she is healthy. None of my patients has ever had a previous heart attack, less than 1% is diabetic or treated with either high blood pressure or cholesterol lowering medications, and less than 5% are obese (BMI>30%) or are past/current smokers.

In distinct contrast, most of the Women's Health Initiative hormone studies participants were many years past their window of opportunity for protection against heart attacks. They were too old, with an average age of 63 (50-79 years) when they initiated their estrogen or estrogen plus progestin. In addition, their lifestyle and general health put them at an increased risk of heart attack or a repeated heart attack. Nearly all of them, some 85%, failed to have significant menopausal symptoms, and finally, they were extremely unhealthy and were already at a high risk for heart attacks.

Remember that about a third of the participants of the Women's Health Initiative Premarin and Prempro Clinical Trials were also included in the Women's Health Initiative Diet Modification Study. All of the women recruited for the Women's Health Initiative Diet Modification Study had to be eating a high fat diet of at least 32% fat calories per day in order for them to participate. Many were obese, some weighing 300 pounds or more. And these obese, unhealthy women comprised nearly a third of the Women's Health Initiative Premarin and Prempro Clinical Trial participants. We all know that many studies have shown that both eating foods that are high in fat and being overweight have a direct increased risk of heart attack and death from heart attack. So these Women's Health Initiative Premarin and Prempro participants were already at a higher risk for heart attack! And remember, the Women's Health Initiative Premarin and Prempro Clinical Trials were primarily designed to look at how estrogen or estrogen plus progestin helped protect against heart attack.

ONLY ONE VARIABLE AT A TIME

You already know rule number one of research is that you never, ever introduce more than one variable into a study, because multiple variables can impact the results. Just like the toddler and the herbal tea, you never know which variable is the one that made the difference. I believe that by studying obese, unhealthy, older, asymptomatic participants, many who were starting their estrogen or estrogen plus progestin years past their "window of opportunity" to prevent heart attack, fatally flawed the results of the Women's Health Initiative Premarin and Prempro Clinical Trials. That means any information we are given about heart attacks from The Women's Health Initiative Premarin and Prempro Clinical Trials data should be examined extremely carefully. We need to put the content of the research data into its proper context.

UNFOUNDED FEARS: 50,000 NEEDLESS DEATHS

Both Women's Health Initiative Estrogen and Estrogen Plus Progestin Observational Studies, the long-term sister studies to the Premarin and Prempro Clinical Studies, indicate that when healthy, symptomatic menopausal women initiate estrogen only or estrogen plus progestin at the usual time, before or within that five year window of opportunity after menopause, for the usual reason, to manage their menopausal symptoms, we see a reduced risk for heart attack (13 and 8 fewer per 10,000 women per year, respectively). So post-menopausal women who initiate their estrogen or estrogen plus progestin before or within the five year window of opportunity and continue it, are protected against future heart attack. That is important life-saving information Dr. Philip Sarrel, emeritus professor in the Departments of Obstetrics, Gynecology & Reproductive Sciences, and Psychology at the Yale School of Medicine wants you to have.

In July 2013, Dr. Sarrel published an article in the American Journal of Public Health that was quickly picked up by the national media. According to Dr. Sarrel and his research team, in the 10-year period from 2002 through 2011 some 50,000 post-menopausal women died prematurely. These were menopausal women who were frightened by the results of the Women's Health Initiative Prempro Clinical trial and either stopped their estrogen therapy or never started estrogen therapy. Fifty thousand dead women. That's as many Americans as were killed in the Vietnam War. Dr. Sarrel said in a video interview, "None of these women lived to be 70 years old. They were all women aged 50-59 who would have used estrogen but did not use it" because of unfounded fears created by the Women's Health Initiative Prempro Clinical Trial.

NEEDLESS DEATH TOLL EXPECTED TO TRIPLE

I met with Dr. Sarrel in my office a few weeks before the publication of his findings, and he confided to me that he believed his statistics were very conservative, and that the number of women who would needlessly die prematurely would actually triple in the next decade to 150,000 because even today, women are still afraid of estrogen. We also discussed the fact that there are many other negative side effects related to stopping estrogen therapy cold turkey which are much more difficult to study or quantify, such as depression, anxiety, migraines, sleeplessness, loss of jobs, or divorce. Even more disturbing? Dr. Sarrel's study only covered post-menopausal women 50-59 years who had a previous hysterectomy, a very small percent of the millions of post- menopausal women who are estimated to have stopped their estrogen therapy because of the Women's Health Initiative's announcement and the media blitz that followed.

Bottom line? I believe, and Dr. Sarrel believes, that women who would have been protected by estrogen died needlessly of heart-related issues because of the misinformation that began with the July 9, 2002 announcement by the Women's Health Initiative's premature termination of the Prempro clinical trial.

RISKS AND BENEFITS

I don't think any researcher or doctor would argue that the benefits outweigh the risks for young, healthy symptomatic women to initiate estrogen therapy, especially if they are pre-menopausal or within five years of menopause, or even under 60 years of age. But some of my patients have asked me if they take the estrogen now, will it put them at increased risk in the future? I believe that the most important statistic from the Women's Health Initiative has to do with longevity.

What we can now tell you is that in both the Women's Health Initiative Premarin and Prempro Clinical Hormone trials, for women who initiated their hormones before age 60 the death rate actually decreased by 30 %. In fact, all four Women's Health Initiative Post-menopausal

Hormone Studies independently demonstrated that hormone users lived longer lives than women who took the placebo.

Estrogen protects a woman's overall health status when it's initiated at the proper time to alleviate menopausal symptoms. Period.

Many of my post-menopausal patients elect to continue their individualized, natural biologically identical hormone therapy for many years to prevent mid-and late post-menopausal conditions. In doing so, I maintain each woman's quality of life as I attempt to protect her against premature death, heart disease, stroke, osteoporosis and fractures, Alzheimer's disease, type 2 diabetes, and colorectal cancer. I have never had a patient have a hip fracture, heart attack, stroke, or colorectal cancer in my clinical practice. In more than 30 years, I have had fewer than 10 patients die from all causes of death, including motor vehicle accidents. I am not aware of anyone who has developed Alzheimer's Disease with early and long-term continued use of estrogen.

I encourage my patients to gradually taper the doses of their hormones slowly and minimally as they age and their metabolism declines. This will reduce the risk of their having significant withdrawal symptoms as they adapt to the lower doses needed to prevent mid- to late-menopausal conditions. As they attempt to reduce their hormone doses as they age, their gauge is to never compromise the quality of their lives.

I believe using hormones, estrogen alone, estrogen plus natural progesterone, and testosterone will not only improve your quality of life, they will increase your longevity and improve your overall outlook on life. That's why I plan to continue symptomatic post-menopausal women on bio-identical estrogen, and estrogen plus progesterone and testosterone therapies obtained from natural vegetable sources for LIFE.

This is similar to what any physician would do for anyone with any other endocrine deficiencies, insulin for diabetes, or thyroid replacement for individuals with low thyroid. All it takes is to try and reduce the estrogen dosage every few years to account for the decreased metabolism that occurs with aging. My patients on hormone replacement are healthy and vibrant as they age gracefully.

Again I emphasize that I include testosterone (the so-called "male hormone") as a key component of a female's hormone therapy. I believe testosterone is a very important ingredient in a woman's quality of life. I always include it as a recommended part of each woman's hormone therapy, even though, incredibly, the FDA currently does not approve any form of testosterone replacement for women. Note, however, the FDA has already approved every form of testosterone replacement for men, in doses that are 15 to 30 times that which I prescribe for my female patients. This makes absolutely no sense to me in the 21st Century.

Perhaps another reason my patients have fewer medical incidents than the women of the Women's health Initiative Premarin and Prempro Clinical Trials is that women on any form of testosterone replacement were excluded from both studies.

FOLLOW THE MONEY

It's important to note that today, the funding for most medical research and education comes from drug companies. Their primary intention is to make and publicize drugs that generate profits, so they may not be the best place from which to gather your healthcare information. You really can't believe everything you read or see on television.

Be aware that phrases like "there is no evidence that this is effective" or "there is no statistical correlation between these things." These statements may simply mean that no research studies have ever been done. It may have been because no one thought that there would be any profit in the research results, so they didn't fund them. That doesn't mean that the treatment should be discounted or dismissed.

ESTROGEN AFTER BREAST CANCER

I have started dozens of selected women on estrogen and testosterone or estrogen, testosterone plus natural progesterone after a diagnosis of breast cancer. I usually consult with and have a breast cancer specialist's OK before I begin this therapy. However, in the interest of being transparent, in my 35 years of practice and 15,000 patients, I have only had two patients in my practice who have died from breast cancer.

IS IT SAFE FOR ME TO START ESTROGEN THERAPY?

I know that women who now understand the truth about estrogen and who have stopped their hormones because of the confusion of the Women's Health Initiative announcement may want to revisit estrogen therapy. To these women, I say I think that's a likely possibility, especially if you're symptomatic, under 60 years of age, within 10 years of menopause and you're healthy. This illustration summarizes the WHI Premarin Clinical Trial for Premarin .625 mg administered orally to post-menopausal women aged 50-79 years and you can easily see that initiating Premarin after the age of 70, estrogen therapy is unsafe. However, lower doses of **non-oral, bio-identical estrogen replacement therapy** may be safe, and improve your low-estrogen physical, emotional, and cognitive menopausal symptoms. Long term

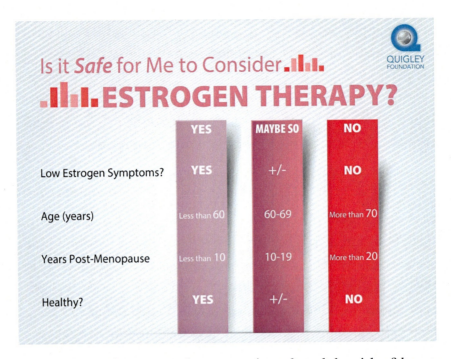

Is it *Safe* for Me to Consider.**ılıl.**
.ılıl.ESTROGEN THERAPY?

	YES	MAYBE SO	NO
Low Estrogen Symptoms?	YES	+/-	NO
Age (years)	Less than 60	60-69	More than 70
Years Post-Menopause	Less than 10	10-19	More than 20
Healthy?	YES	+/-	NO

use of estrogen and estrogen plus progestin reduced the risk of heart attack and premature, needless deaths in women. Recent research has shown that the use of the natural progesterone markedly reduces the risk of invasive breast cancer seen with more than five years of use of synthetic progestins.

I've had a very comfortable experience with my natural estrogen patch and testosterone and progesterone creams. Being able to regulate my hormones by listening to my own body's needs and not being dictated to conform with medicine's "norm" appears to be the only sane approach to hormone replacement for me. Prior to the natural creams and the estrogen patch, I could not create a steady, even-keel consistency in my hormone levels, and thus, my life experience. Now I control my experience by listening to and feeling my own needs. Then, I adjust my hormones accordingly. Isn't this what real medicine is supposed to be?

Carolina

Chapter 10

Putting It All Together

People are like stained-glass windows. They sparkle and shine when the sun is out, but when the darkness sets in, their true beauty is revealed only if there is a light from within.

Elizabeth Kubler-Ross

CREATING BALANCE

I have seen that the right dosages of replacement hormones creates the physical, emotional, and spiritual balance necessary to live your best life. I know that once you find your correct hormonal zone, you'll begin to find real balance in your life, too. I prefer to use these natural bio-identical hormones, rather than synthetic ones for estrogen therapy because:

- They are not modified solely so that they can be patented.

- A single, simple blood test can be done at any commercial laboratory, as a safety net, to determine if you are receiving "too much" or "too little" of that hormone.

I have found the estrogen patch, cream or gel to be, in most cases, the most effective and efficient form of estrogen therapy delivery because:

- It is 100 percent natural.

- Lower doses have the same effect as higher doses of oral estrogen therapy.

- The estrogen patch provides the steadiest and most stable release of estradiol delivery both for relief of symptoms and accurate blood estradiol determinations.

- You can fine-tune your estrogen by cutting the patch and adding or subtracting from your usual dosage of estrogen cream or gel as you and your doctor deem necessary.

Most of the typical menopausal symptoms are related to estrogen deficiency and are reversed by estrogen therapy, which is why estrogen is the first hormone I usually replace. Testosterone is a feel good bonus many women say they can't do without. Progesterone is recommended primarily to protect against the endometrial cancer of the uterus, but remember, the most commonly used synthetic form of progestin, Provera, was implicated as an increased risk factor for both breast cancer and heart disease in the Women's Health Initiative Prempro Clinical Trials in 2002. I do not prescribe Provera for my patients.

BENEFITS OF TRANSDERMAL DELIVERY

Estrogen is metabolized primarily in the liver, so when it is taken in oral pill form, more than 90 percent will be metabolized before ever reaching your general blood circulation. Oral estrogen is an inefficient hormone delivery system. The estrogen patch, cream, or gel, however, delivers estradiol directly into the general blood circulation, by-passing the liver. This more closely mimics the normal ovarian estrogen, which is directly released into your general blood circulation so it can be delivered to every cell of your body.

In my own practice, I have seen a 300-fold difference in the amount of estrogen needed by different women to alleviate their symptoms. That difference can be exaggerated by an individual's lifestyle in the following ways:

1. METABOLISM. If you are a younger woman, as well as one who exercises frequently, you will generally metabolize estrogen faster and require more estrogen than older, less active women. As women age their metabolism slows down. This is the reason why women who have been on estrogen or estrogen plus progesterone therapy for several years may be able to reduce their dosage of estrogen as they age without affecting the quality of their life.

2. WEIGHT. If you are overweight, you may require larger doses than smaller women. However, fat tissue produces estrogen (estrone). This probably explains why obese women have fewer menopausal symptoms compared to those with low body fat.

3. ACTIVITY LEVEL. If you are highly active, you will tend to metabolize estrogen more rapidly than inactive women and may require larger doses of estrogen replacement. That means if you exercise or start

exercising more, you will likely require higher doses of estrogen replacement.

4. DOSES OF HORMONES AND OTHER MEDICATIONS. If you are very sensitive to other medications, if you require one-quarter to one-half the usual adult dose of other medications, then you will most likely require lower doses of estrogen as well. However, if you require more than the usual amount of other medications, implying that you have a higher metabolism, you may also require higher doses of estrogen. In addition, if you require higher than average dosage of estrogen, you will probably require higher than average dosage of testosterone, too. Also, it is my clinical impression that changes of doses of the various SSRI antidepressants, such as Prozac, Zoloft, and Wellbutrin, may affect estradiol activity. Starting, stopping, or modifying the doses of SSRIs appears to modify serum estradiol activity, so if you have recently modified the dosage of your antidepressant, you may need to modify your dosage of hormones in order to remain in your estrogen zone.

MY METHODOLOGY

As I initiate estrogen replacement, I tend to start with a dose that is lower than what I feel is the optimum dose needed for each patient. It's that shower thing again, I'm trying to make sure the hormone dose is *just right* for that individual. If the hormone dose is too "hot" or too much, then we need to back off. If it's too "cold" or not enough, we need to add more. This helps to ensure that we determine the optimal lowest dosage for each individual hormone for each unique woman.

Here's something you should know. I find that the first symptoms to improve are often the physical symptoms, such as the hot flashes, night sweats, palpitations, and sleep disturbances, but I notice that a higher level of estrogen replacement is often needed to improve the psychological or emotional symptoms, such as anxiety, irritability, moodiness, and depression. It is not uncommon to discover that even higher amounts of estrogen are needed to stabilize the cognitive changes, including the problems with concentration, short-term memory, and forgetfulness. I find that these early post-menopausal physical, psychological, and cognitive symptoms are usually reversed within 48 hours of initiation of the correct amount of estrogen replacement when you monitor your progress on the Women's Awareness Calendar.

If you have bladder and vaginal atrophy or thinning, it will take a bit longer, usually two to six weeks, for your body to respond to the correct amount of estrogen replacement. The reason for this is that the growth of new vaginal and bladder tissue, which is stimulated by estrogen, is needed to increase the thickness of these specific tissues in order for these symptoms to be reversed.

Having the ability to monitor my own body and its response to hormone replacement gives me a much improved outlook on my health and aging. I feel that I am better able to respond to the nuances of change that occur in response to exercise and stress and my mood is much more optimistic! While many people would not expect age to bring positive experiences, in fact, it does! As responsibilities to children and family decrease, I have enjoyed a new understanding of and relationship with myself and life. Take time to know yourself, it is a great gift.

Jeanette

Chapter 11

Finding the Right Medical Partner

You take your life in your own hands, and what happens? A terrible thing: no one to blame.

Erica Jong

LISTEN TO YOUR INNER VOICE!

So you're educated about what really happened with the Women's Health Initiative. You've used the Women's Awareness Calendar, and you've tracked your symptoms. You're convinced that non-oral, individualized, bio-identical hormone replacement is the right path for you, and you're ready to find a healthcare provider who will work with you. Terrific!

One of the benefits of hormone replacement therapy is that you'll begin to feel like yourself again. Many of my patients say that is the first domino of the physical, emotional, and spiritual growth that accompanies the wisdom of menopause. One of the first signposts of that domino is listening to your inner voice. That voice is wise, that voice is knowing, and that voice is you. It's the voice you can and should use when discussing your health with your doctor.

Your insight, your "knowing" gives your doctor important clues about what's going on with you not just physically, but emotionally, cognitively, and spiritually. Your doctor's insight, that is, his or her belief system, is going to influence how he or she treats you. For instance, if your doctor believes in synthetic hormones, and you prefer natural, bio-identical hormones, that's an important conversation to have, and it could be one that actually ends your relationship with that doctor.

Many women make the mistake of being loyal to the doctor who delivered their babies, or who helped them with a previous health issue. Loyalty is a wonderful virtue, but not if it means sacrificing your health. So that's why it's important to find a doctor you are comfortable with, and one who is in alignment with your beliefs, and is the right practitioner for you.

AWARENESS: IT'S TIME TO SEE A DOCTOR

Your body is changing, you feel different, and you're listening to your inner voice, so you know something is "off" and it's time to seek professional help. Wonderful! You're on a journey that begins with a quest to feel better, and I believe that awareness is the first step in the healing process. You have everything in you at this moment to heal. Finding the right practitioner can act as a catalyst, speeding up that process. In fact, I believe you are already healing, simply by asking for that guidance.

My experience has been that once you put your attention on your health, things begin to change, so it's absolutely critical that you are completely comfortable and honest with yourself and your physician or healthcare provider. That's why I encourage you to look around and find a medical practitioner who is right for you. This is someone who you will be talking to about very intimate details of your life, and everyone has different comfort levels when it comes to that kind of communication. I once worked with a truly brilliant physician whose bedside manner was atrocious, but whose credentials and skills were impeccable. Some women loved him, because he was a straight talker who was all business. Others refused to see him for the same reasons. So finding the right healthcare provider, someone who "speaks your language" and can work with you, is critical.

YOUR LIFESTYLE AFFECTS YOUR HEALTH

Remember, your inner knowingness alerts you that something is "off", so I am convinced that the same inner knowingness can be accessed for healing. My decades of experience tell me that you know your body better than any medical practitioner. What's more, I believe you should come to that first appointment prepared to spend some time getting to know each other, kind of like a first date. So be prepared to tell your doctor about not only your health issues, but also about what's going on in your life and about your lifestyle. For instance, what kind of a diet do you have, how much alcohol do you drink, are you a smoker, do you exercise regularly? Are you stressed at work? Do you have family issues or aging parents? The doctor or healthcare practitioner must look at your whole life, because our bodies often physically reflect our emotional environment. So it may be that by only treating the physical issues, the emotional triggers or issues remain untouched and still need to be addressed. That's important life-work that you'll need to do in order to completely heal. However, since it's work that's done outside of the doctor's office, I believe a follow up visit is critically important, even if your health concerns have been solved. It gives you and your doctor a metric, a line with which we can measure your health and healing progress. It also gives you feedback, information that you can use as you become more aware of yourself, of your body and your inner voice.

RESEARCH AND ASK AROUND

Women talk to each other. A lot. Women are amazing resources for each other, especially when it comes to their unique issues like periods, pregnancy and menopause. I've seen that women share this kind of personal information with each other readily, that they communicate easily and support each other regularly. A first step for you as you research your options would be to talk to your friends, your sister(s) or your mother - someone you trust and have confidence in. Get a feel for what their menopausal medical experiences have been, who they consider experts, and why. Then go on a fact-finding mission of your own. Use the internet, research, and find a doctor or nurse practitioner who feels right to you. Check out his or her background, education, credentials, and affiliations. So many people use social media sites, you may be able to get a feel for his or her personality by the posts or pictures they include. Is this someone you feel you can talk to? Someone you would want to spend time with? Is this the right person to trust with your health questions? These are all important things to know before you even make an appointment. And when you do call, what's the vibe you get from the office? Is the person who answers the phone helpful, or in a hurry? Does it feel like you are important, or that you're a number? Trust your inner knowingness and make a decision based on what you feel. This may not be the right doctor or office for you, and you may know it just from that first phone call.

PREPARING FOR THE FIRST APPOINTMENT

If you do decide to make that first appointment, make sure you do everything you can to prepare for it. Ask if there is anything specific that you can do now so that the scheduled time with your doctor is as efficient and productive as possible. Is there paperwork that you can fill out at home or ahead of time? Can the paperwork be emailed or faxed? What do you need to bring with you to your first appointment? Drivers license? Will you need medical insurance information or a medical card? What is the estimated length of time you'll be seen, and what are the charges? Are you expected to pay anything at the time of the visit; is there a copay? Is there parking available? What, if any, are the costs for parking? The more you prepare, the more work you do ahead of time, the more productive your appointment will be, so if time is limited you'll be able to make the most of it. You'll be ready to inform the doctor about what has and what has not been working in your life. Since many times our health is affected by our daily routines, it's important to communicate what's going on with you. Do you have a diet and exercise routine? Do you take any vitamins or prescriptions? What is your family and work life like? What are the stressors in your life and how have you been dealing with them? Are there major life changes taking place right now for you? I suggest you write these things down in a notebook, and bring that notebook with you to your appointment. That way you can not only inform your doctor about what's going on, you can also take notes during your time with him or her, and keep track of your progress.

If you are transparent and specific about your life choices as well as what you are seeking and asking for help with, you're going to feel very vulnerable. That's because you are literally opening and exposing yourself to someone who is a stranger. But remember to leave your pride at the door and come into the appointment knowing it is a safe space. You deserve to live your best life and your doctor can be a catalyst for your process of self discovery and self healing... after all your body is your vehicle on your journey and adventure of life! Love yourself enough to be honest with your doctor in order to receive your best treatment.

TIME WELL SPENT

That first appointment is the foundation of your relationship with your doctor, so trust that first impression. The most important thing is to see and feel if your doctor resonates with you, speaks your language, understands your life and your lifestyle. Why? Your doctor is someone you will most likely be spending time with over the next few years, so it is important that the two of you get along and are on the same page with regard to your health. I believe it's important to recognize that this is a relationship, so like all relationships, you should both take a little bit of time to get to know each other in the beginning. You have already done your homework, so you know a little about his or her background, but now it's time to communicate face to face with your doctor. By setting a tone and dialogue now, you and your doctor are creating a foundation of a mutually equal and balanced relationship and that can prevent problems from arising in the future. It's very important to spend extra time at that first appointment getting to know each other. I would suggest spending at least a half hour at that first appointment. I personally have always set aside a full hour for each of my new patients, and it's something I have found to be beneficial for both of us.

TIMING IS EVERYTHING

I believe one of the biggest tragedies in medicine is that the patient and the practitioner are not present with one another during the appointment. Let me explain. The "old school" patient and doctor relationship meant a busy waiting room with lots of patients, busy examining rooms and very little one on one time with each other. The perception is that this is a busy doctor, so he or she must be a good doctor.

You've probably had this experience; you make an appointment with a busy doctor hoping for excellent care.

But the doctor is busy because appointments are often double booked, so the doctor falls behind and spends much of the day running late, quickly seeing as many patients as possible, all the while making snap decisions based on cursory examinations. That means when it's your turn to be examined, you, too are quickly diagnosed. The doctor wasn't really present; he or she was thinking about the other examining rooms filled with patients. You were likely not present either, feeling frustrated because of the long wait, and rushed when the doctor finally entered. But, since doctors are perceived as God-like, all knowing experts, most patients don't question his or her nearly instant diagnosis.

I can tell you that unless you make sure your appointment is either the first or last of the day, you may end up getting less out of your visit than you might have hoped.

Remember this is a collaborative relationship based on your health. Your doctor depends on you for information about how and what your body is feeling. You depend on your doctor for his or her skill, knowledge, experience and recommendations in order for you to make an informed decision. Decide upon a plan that works both from a medical standpoint and from your lifestyle standpoint.

WHAT TO BRING TO THE FIRST APPOINTMENT

I encourage you to come to that first appointment with your Women's Awareness Calendar, filled in and full of information about your symptoms from the past month or two, and information about your life including a clear, concise description of your symptoms (in fact I would even recommend that you write a brief paragraph of your health history) and a list of questions.

The Women's Awareness Calendar is more than a snapshot, it's a monthly "movie" of your hormonal health; that is invaluable to you and your doctor. A doctor's office can be intimidating, you may feel rushed, so having your clear, concise history and your list of questions ready means you'll get answers immediately. What's more, some of those questions may trigger additional questions, by you or by your doctor. It's critical that you have an open flow of communication.

I am a doctor, and have my field of expertise, but we are still both human beings. I have seen all too often that patients make the mistake of giving their power away to their doctors, and not listening to their own powerful inner voice, instead of relying on a quick diagnosis from a busy physician. I believe that is a mistake. You must assume full responsibility for your health. Seek a medical professional who is willing to take the time to listen to you, and to work with you as you begin your Hormone

Replacement Therapy. If your appointment with your doctor didn't feel right, if something felt off, or if you didn't feel like you were being heard or your opinion was not acknowledged, if you were constantly interrupted, would you want to see that person again? Probably not.

MAKE SURE YOU ARE HEARD

Pay special attention to interruptions by your doctor. Research shows that the average doctor interrupts his or her patient within 12 seconds of an office visit. Does your doctor listen or interrupt? Is he or she open to your questions, or do you feel rushed? If you're comfortable, if this seems like a relationship you want to pursue, a person you can trust with very intimate details of your life, then set up your next appointment. Ask when it would be a good time for a follow up appointment, and make that appointment before you leave the office.

PLAN YOUR GOOD HEALTH

Work with your doctor to create an individualized plan for your health. This plan is not rigid, but is adaptable; it can and should be modified as your life flows and changes. Start modifying your life with what you feel you need to change first. For instance, if part of your plan is to eat less sugar and more fresh fruits and vegetables, then a subsequent visit to your healthcare provider may show you've lost weight and lowered your blood pressure. You may now want to adjust your plan to also include walking or exercising for 15 minutes to 30 minutes at least three to five times a week.

Again, this is an opportunity for learning and creating awareness about your body and its needs. A good plan facilitates change and means a better, more fulfilled, healthier life.

I believe that you are responsible for your own body and health. As a physician, my job is to guide you into making the best possible choices you can make in and outside of my office. I can tell you it's important to drink up to eight glasses of water every day, but it's up to you to fill those glasses and drink them. If you're only going to drink four glasses per day, that's something you need to communicate to me: it helps me to understand what's going on with your body and why.

FOLLOW UP

I personally see most of my patients every two weeks until we have a clear or empty Women's Awareness Calendar. This typically means an initial visit plus three or four subsequent appointments to determine your individualized estrogen, testosterone, and progesterone zones. And of course, what you do outside of my office is the most important factor when it comes to your good health. How often are you seen for follow up visits? As often as you feel it is beneficial to you. If you feel you need to come in every week initially, you need to let your doctor know. Remember your inner knowingness.

I believe that after any medical appointment we also have "life-work" to do in preparation for the next visit. Just like children have homework when they get home from school to practice what they have learned, this lifework will help you to learn about, and to create awareness about yourself and your body's patterns.

Your life-work is a daily practice, and just like you keep track of what's going on with you physically with the Women's Awareness Calendar, I invite you to also keep track of what's going on with you emotionally by journaling. When you keep a written record of what's going on in your life and compare it to what's going on in your body, you and your doctor will be able to see patterns, and that's important information about how you react to your life's stresses and joys. What's more, there are benefits of body awareness and monitoring. We all have "off" days, but if something bigger is going on, your inner knowingness, combined with the documentation from the Women's Awareness Calendar and your journal will help you and your doctor to work together to solve the problem.

A PERSONAL OBSERVATION

After practicing medicine for decades and meeting countless healthcare professionals, doctors, nurses, and nurse practitioners, I can tell you that many of these wonderful healers began medical careers because they were curious about the human body and how it functions, but that, like me, they were also answering a call to serve.

Most doctors want to be of service, choosing to spend their time, energy, and resources to pass on and teach their experience, maybe even possibly furthering the understanding in a specific field or branch in medicine. I believe being a doctor is an ongoing learning process, and many of my colleagues feel the same way. Although school taught us the basics of our education and specialization, we have learned far more throughout the years from our patients, so whether it's giving a patient a specific hormone, listening to them so they feel heard and understood, or giving them information to make informed decisions for themselves, a wise doctor is always open to listening, learning, and growing.

A true healer is someone who creates a comfortable, nurturing environment that makes it safe for healing to occur.

Chapter 12

The WOW Factor

Our deepest fear is not that we are inadequate. Our deepest fear is that we are powerful beyond measure.

It is our light, not our darkness that most frightens us.

We ask ourselves "Who am I to be brilliant, gorgeous, talented, fabulous?" Actually, who are you not to be? You are a child of God.

Your playing small does not serve the world. There's nothing enlightened about shrinking so that other people won't feel insecure around you.

We are all meant to shine, as children do. We were born to make manifest the glory of God that is within us.

It's not just in some of us; it is in everyone, and as we let our own light shine, we unconsciously give other people permission to do the same. As we're liberated from our own fear, our presence automatically liberates others.

Marianne Williamson

Have you ever noticed a woman who walks into a room and seems to be "glowing"? There is something different about her, an inner light, and it is almost indescribable. It's as if she is shining from within. The light flows though her eyes and her very being and her vibrant presence is known and felt by all. She is strong, confident, and gracious. She is present, aware, acts deliberately and is "on purpose." You may think it is her external beauty that attracts but it is her internal beauty that is shining though, that gives her what I call the WOW Factor!

For years I have had a photograph of my three beautiful daughters on the desk of my office. That's not just a father's pride. Many of my patients comment on the picture and say how beautiful each of my daughters is. I always thank them for their comments, but add quite proudly that it is the inner beauty of each of my children that is truly amazing. Their internal beauty shines through and simply eclipses the physical.

So many of us have grown accustomed to living a stressful lifestyle that leaves us feeling unfulfilled, unhappy, powerless, and almost completely disconnected from our true, beautiful essence. That inner light dulls, as our chaotic, deadline oriented, pressure-filled world programs us to seek answers externally, or to value things that have no real value, like the kind of clothes we wear and the cars we drive. Those are things society values, but they do not feed the soul, they do not give lasting joy, or tap into the vast power that is within each of us. Instead of looking to others for their approval and power, I believe it's very important instead to look within and to embrace the power that is already always within each of us.

YOU'VE GOT THE POWER!

Hormone Replacement Therapy can help a woman get in tune with her body and discover her individualized ideal/optimal hormonal zones, which helps her rebalance her internal system, and once balanced, she is able to approach her world differently. It's that difference in perspective that is such an integral part of the WOW Factor. You are much more powerful than you realize, and if you listen, you will always know from deep within your soul what is true, what is right, and what to do in any situation. And when you are in tuned with your "True Self", WOW! Your world just seems to flow with positive energy. I know it, because I see it and experience this beautiful change with my patients every single day.

So what do I mean by listening to and getting in touch with your "True Self"? Here's an example you can probably relate to. As a mother you don't need a degree in medicine to know when your child is sick. You have an intuitive state of knowingness about your child's health. It would not matter if the most respected pediatrician in the world tried to tell you that your child was okay. If you knew your child was sick, then in all likelihood, your child really was sick. You would continue to pursue getting the necessary help for your child, no matter what obstacles were placed on your path. Every mother knows to trust her intuition when it comes to caring for her child. She's listening to her inner voice, she's in touch with her True Self.

Similarly, you have the intuition to instinctively know what is best for you - your body, your mind, and your spirit - and it's as easy as simply listening to your inner voice. The inner voice is not the chatter. Who is observing the chatter? The inner voice is the knowingness behind the chatter. So why not start now? Now is the time to take responsibility to balance and center your Self.

SELF-CENTERED

Here's something to consider. Many of us have developed a programmed thought pattern or belief system that tells us that it is selfish to put our needs first. I don't believe that to be true. I instead prefer the "oxygen mask effect" where parents are told on every airplane that in the case of an emergency, they must put their own oxygen masks on first so they can assist their children with their mask. If you pass out from asphyxiation, how can your child get his or her mask on?

Women especially seem to be programmed to put themselves last and take care of everyone else in their lives first. But in order to be truly be of service to those around you, it is absolutely necessary to be aware of your own needs. That may mean putting yourself first at times. I think that when you let your inner voice lead the way, once you listen to your True Self, just like a mother who knows when her child is sick, you will always make the right decision for yourself and those you love. That internal guidance, your intuition from your heart and soul always has your highest good in mind. If you listen carefully, you may hear your heart and soul tell you that it is OK to take care of yourself first, something that's very difficult for so many women.

CREATING BALANCE AND CHANGE

Think about it. When you are centered and balanced, and able to contribute to the world around you simply by living by example, you create a ripple effect that is more powerful than you could ever imagine. When you change, those around you change. As you develop into the newest and best version of you, those around you pick up your shift in energy. They too feel empowered to choose what is in alignment with their higher Self, just like you are making that choice. It's an energy shift that is tangible, and it's an energy shift that creates tangible results.

THE WOW FACTOR

The key to becoming all that you can be right now is what I call the WOW factor and I believe it can be a tremendous tool for you to use as you balance your body, mind, and spirit. I believe WOW stands for Wellness, Oneness, and Wholeness. Every one of us can benefit from living a WOW life, one that is balanced and aligned, filled with love and compassion. It's easy and will help ensure your life is filled with incredible, unlimited potential. And it begins with awareness. Whether it's balancing your hormones, or balancing kids and career, it all begins with an awareness of what your life is, and what your life can be.

EASE OR DISEASE?

I believe that wellness is a deliberate, ongoing choice. Wellness is a view of health that emphasizes the state of balance of your entire being and its ongoing development. In contrast, Western medicine is instead focused on illness or "dis-ease" - what is out of balance. I believe it's much more important to be proactive about our health and ease instead into balance, alignment and wellness.

Think about wellness for your body or caring for your body in the same way you care for your car. Your car needs to be maintained in order to operate to its fullest ability, and so does your body. I believe life is the journey, not the destination. So make sure to fill your tank with fuel and get those periodic check ups. When you're tuned up and well maintained, you are ready to go no matter where life takes you. And when you self-maintain, just like the parent on an airplane with the oxygen mask, you are being of service to all. If you do not maintain yourself, if you run out of energy or fuel, just like a car, you will break down and be of service to no one. So how you take care of yourself matters.

BACK TO THE BASICS

I know doctors who stress the importance of clean fresh water, a balanced diet and plenty of exercise. What you put into your body, your fuel, is critical, and how you use that fuel is also critical. It's all about input, and output. If you eat too much and don't exercise enough your body stores fat and you gain weight. But I'm going to take it a step further and tell you that while diet and exercise are both important, so is a good night's sleep, the way you breathe, and the water you drink. You can only live for three minutes without oxygen, so your survival depends primarily on your breath, and your breath is an excellent indication of the state of the health of your body. A ten minute drive on the freeway during rush hour and you're likely to start breathing more quickly and shallowly. That's because you're in a situation that your body recognizes as stressful, so it releases what it believes to be the appropriate hormonal response. Your body tenses, your senses are on heightened alert, your heart rate and blood pressure increase, and non-essential systems like your digestive and immune system are shut down. Your brain is focused on danger, so it is looking for the source of the threat in a "big picture" manner and that may mean you have difficulty focusing on small tasks. And since most of us take two or more of these rush hour trips per day, they're taking a toll on us, creating a chemical chain reaction of stress hormones in our bodies that makes it really difficult for us to stay balanced and healthy. I personally have found that my morning commute is the most stressful time in my day. So a year ago I started taking slow, deep deliberate breaths as I drove to work, and the result has been that I feel energized and really ready to work when I arrive at the office.

TAKE FIVE BREATHS PER MINUTE

Being conscious of your breathing, slowing it down with deeper, slower and steady breaths can actually lower your blood pressure, your heart rate, and your stress hormones. The optimal rhythm to achieve balance of your peripheral nervous systems, is to inhale slowly and steadily for six seconds and then to exhale slowly and steadily for six seconds, or to take 5 breaths per minute. Try it for just a few minutes and you'll see results almost immediately. The best part? It's completely free, you can do it anywhere, and in front of anybody! I recommend you use this technique in any stressful situation, but know it is especially valuable when you're going for a job interview, when you have difficult conversations with a loved one, or during one of those memorable holiday family gatherings.

FROM WATER COMES LIFE

You are mostly made of water and that means water is used by every cell, every organ, every part of you. Water regulates your body temperature, and moves nutrients throughout your cells; your bones have less water than your brain, but your blood is almost all water. In fact, the average adult body is made of about 70% water. Here's something you may find very interesting. Water makes up as much as 75% of a newborn infant's body weight, and some obese adults have as little as 45% water by weight. So drinking enough water and drinking the right kind of water is key to your health. I tell my patients to drink at least six to ten eight-ounce glasses of water every day to ensure you are flushing toxins and waste from your body, and optimally that water should be purified or distilled, clean and fresh.

FOOD AS FUEL

Fresh food is also essential to good health. The more nutritionally packed food you include every single day, the healthier you will become. Food is more than fuel, it's medicine for your body and can actually help to repair your body from the inside out. Your optimal diet is a rainbow mix of carbohydrates, fats, proteins and micronutrients, but the amount you need actually decreases as you age.

A 30 year old woman needs about 2000 calories a day for optimum health, but a 50 year old woman needs only about 1600 calories a day. In all cases, your diet should include organic, fresh unprocessed fruits and vegetables, as well as Certified Drug Free protein rich legumes, meat, poultry, and fish. You should avoid all hormone and drug-ingested meats and dairy foods, as well as all processed and junk foods. Processed foods tend to decrease the fiber, increase the salt, and increase the Glycemic Index of the food.

The Glycemic Index is a measurement carried out on carbohydrate-containing foods and their impact on our blood sugar. Glycemic Index is a relatively new way of analyzing foods. High Glycemic Index foods, like junk food, fast food, sugary candy and cookies, result in a fast, high blood sugar rise, causing a strong burst of insulin to be released into your bloodstream. This has a major consequence on your body's chemistry,; as you know, insulin is a hormone and as a hormone it is created by the pancreas, but used by virtually every other cell in your body.

In contrast, eating foods that are low on the glycemic index, like fresh fruits and vegetables, doesn't produce that fast, high sugar rise, that roller coaster ride of intense energy followed by intense lethargy. Instead of causing a release of insulin, eating the right combination of low glycemic index carbohydrates, high fiber foods, lean protein and "good" fats, provides a slower, more sustained, balanced release of glucagon. Glucagon breaks down fat and causes your blood cells to dilate, so your body has more oxygen and can burn even more fat. It's a win/win situation. Simply by choosing the right foods, you can get those foods to work with your body to burn fat.

TAKE YOUR VITAMINS

You should also consider supplementing your diet with vitamins, the micronutrients so important for health and growth. Vitamins such as B and C are water soluble, and help to regulate your metabolism. These vitamins are important in the processing of carbohydrates, fats, and proteins into energy. Vitamin C plays a critical role in your body's defense mechanism, helping to maintain, clear and clean blood vessels. I think it's important for vegetarians to know that vitamin B12 is only found in foods of animal origin, so they may be deficient in that important micronutrient. If you're a vegetarian or vegan, I recommend either a sublingual or intramuscular dose of B12, because it can markedly enhance many menopausal women's energy and sense of well-being. Again, it's simply making informed, good choices about what you put into your body. But good health is not just about input, it's also about output, or exercise.

YOU GOT TO MOVE IT, MOVE IT!

The American Heart Association recommends getting at least 150 minutes of moderate exercise every week. That breaks down to about a half hour of exercise, five times a week. While it doesn't sound like much, taking 30 minutes out of your day for physical activity will do wonders for your heart, body, and your outlook on life. Exercising on a daily basis in ways that gets your blood pumping will create a positive energy flow throughout your entire body.

I'm not suggesting any kind of radical change in your life. Just taking a brisk walk is heart healthy; in fact, anything that gets your heart pumping and the oxygen flowing in your bloodstream is terrific for your health.

There are lots of ways to get in a little extra exercise. One simple thing I have done my entire life is to take the stairs rather than an elevator for two or three flights. So think about things that you enjoy, that are part of your day, that also increase your heart rate. How about a hike, a swim, a group dance program or even some really good sex? Every one of these activities is good for your heart and your health, and they're also fun.

I'd also like you to consider the fact that osteoporosis, or degenerative bone loss, can be prevented with strength training or weight resistance training. That's why Yoga and Pilates are such good choices for women. They improve balance, strength, and mobility. Use your body and your body weight to build strength in both your muscles and your bones.

Research proves that exercise feels good. When you exercise, your body releases endorphins, or "feel good" hormones. And they're addictive. When you get into the exercise groove, you'll find that you'll want to exercise for longer and more often. Those endorphins are doing their job. Exercise with a friend and you're more likely to stay motivated, and keep up the exercise routine, even on days when you just don't feel like making the effort yourself.

YOUR BODIES

As a physician I recognize that we all have a physical body which requires constant care. I further believe that we also have mental, emotional, and spiritual bodies that need our attention as well, and that's why it's so important to be in balance. I believe each of these bodies is inter-connected to one another, creating a "oneness" within us that makes us whole and balanced. They are a team working together, so if one or more of your "bodies" is off or out of balance, you'll feel off or imbalanced. The menopausal women who come to my office are looking to balance their physical bodies, but the physical lack of hormones also manifests itself in mental anguish; emotional peaks and valleys that can be devastating to a woman's spirit. The good news is that when your four bodies are balanced and aligned, your potential is unlimited. Just like the woman who walks into the room and whom everyone notices, you are positive, glowing and alive. I believe that amazing life force energy is available to you, too. It all begins with awareness.

YOU THINK AND FEEL, THEREFORE YOU ARE

What you think affects you and your body. What you feel also affects you and your body. Your feelings are the best indicators as to what you are to do in any situation and when you tap into that inner knowingness, you'll always do the right thing. So when you feel something, really feel it.

The same way I like to think of your physical body as a car, I think of your emotional body as a stoplight. Do you sense a situation where you see or feel a red light? Stop and feel into it and then decide if you really want to continue moving in the same direction. When you feel a yellow light, proceed with caution; that will serve you best. However, when you feel in your gut that all is well, it's a green light ... go!

What if your feelings are direct signals for your life's journey? You are here to experience a wide range of emotions, but also to neutralize them. Notice people and the things that trigger various emotions. Eliminate or modify your triggers to negative emotions. Defuse the energy around them. Let go of the extremes and find balance by taking responsibility for yourself and your life.

CLEAN UP ON AISLE 6!

We all have a mess or messes in our lives that need to be dealt with. Being aware and connected with our emotions is imperative to notice triggers and see where there is still work to be done in our lives. I call it "Clean up on Aisle 6." But be sure to focus on *your* Aisle 6 cleanup, not everyone else's. If you're focused on everyone else's problems, guess whose never gets solved? Yours. So clean up those lingering emotions right here, right now! It will help balance you emotionally, and help give you patience when others struggle with their own "Clean up on aisle 6."

The sad truth is I see many women in my practice who have talked themselves into believing lies about who they really are. "I'm not worthy," "I'm not good enough," "I'm not pretty enough," "I'm not slim enough," "I'm too old," or "I can't." These are the messages they give themselves over and over again and they're the same excuses that can prevent you from living your best life.

Where focus goes, energy flows. That's how our thoughts, feelings and beliefs create your own reality. You are worthy, you are good enough, and you can do anything you decide to do. But just saying these positive messages or affirmations is not enough. You have to repeat these positive affirmations until you believe them. You do have freedom of choice, and thus control, over the thoughts that you choose to keep and focus your attention on. Reprogram your mind and become a newer, and even more authentic version of your True Self.

DO YOU WANT TO HAVE IT A.L.L.?

I believe there are three key components to living that beautiful, integrated life; they are Authenticity, Love, and Legacy, but everything begins with being true to who you are. As Shakespeare said, "To thine own self be true," so ask yourself. Are you living your life or are you living the life others chose for you?

AUTHENTICITY

Be a first-rate version of yourself, instead of a second-rate version of somebody else.

Judy Garland

Authenticity is the degree to which one is true to one's own personality, spirit, or character despite external pressures. Do you live your own life, or do you live the life that others choose for you? Are you choosing to become the most authentic and best version of yourself? Being authentic means knowing and speaking your truth. I have a patient whose struggle with an advanced cancer was nothing compared to the struggle she faced in her daily life. It was only when she stopped and spoke her truth that her life began to change. She said out loud, "I now choose to make different choices." By remaining strong and consistent, she not only was true to herself, she was able to focus on her disease and really take the journey within, to discover who she really was. I was honored to watch her heal as her inner light began first as a flicker, and then grew to a blinding, beautiful, powerful beam. Her cancer is gone! By being true to herself she healed herself and she became the catalyst that transformed her family into a loving, supportive, and healthy relationship.

LOVE

Love yourself first, and everything else falls into line. You really have to love yourself to get anything done in this world.

Lucille Ball

As humans, I truly believe our natural state of being is love. I say this because, as you know, I have witnessed the miracle of birth thousands of times and every single newborn brings with it into this world a palpable, energetic wave of love. Just watch a mother hold her baby for the first time and you feel overwhelmed by that love. Science can't measure it, but all of us can certainly feel it.

What if you loved yourself as much as a new mother loves her child? How much would it change your world?

Once you experience self love, it allows you to fully express and share that authentic love with others. Self love isn't selfish, it's self-centered and is the highest gift you can give to yourself, as well as others. Love is what defines us as humans. The Beatles really did say it best: *"Love is all you need."* Love just is. It is a feeling. It is a knowing. It is a state of Being. You must be love to experience love. So go within. Divine love really is Divine. Love yourself now. WOW.

LEGACY

If you get, give. If you learn, teach.

Maya Angelou

A Legacy is something left behind that shows the world how you chose to spend time, energy, and resources—an expression of passion in a meaningful and purposeful way. People of all ages have the potential to leave dramatic and long-lasting legacies to future generations, right now. Ghandi said *"Be the change you wish to see in the world."* We are all unique with different strengths, talents, and gifts and when we embrace and express our uniqueness, we can each begin to leave behind a meaningful legacy. That genuine giving connects us to others in a way that is almost unbelievable. The ripples of our kindness reach beyond the boundaries of countries, through generations, and beyond our own lifetimes. Living the good life means sharing your goodness with others.

Menopause can be a time to share your goodness with others as you become the best and most authentic version of yourself, the very best "ME" you can be; that woman who is completely balanced in body, mind, emotions, and spirit. I have seen how beautifully powerful and positive the benefits of that balanced, authentic self can be for all of us when it multiplies and grows. When you tap into that endless, vibrant energy that is the true you, and bring your self, your "ME" and all of your amazing strengths, talents, natural gifts, and experience to the world and then share those positive gifts with all of the others who also have so much to contribute, the other "ME"s come together to form the enormous and powerful collective "WE". And that incredible, positive energy absolutely has the power to not only change individuals, but to also transform the world.

This is why you are here on the earth NOW. We are all currently witnessing the greatest transformation or shift in consciousness that the human race on the planet earth has ever experienced.

As a physician, I know that your sense of self, your belief about who you are, can make or break your physical health. Remember, what you resist will always persist. I know that by focusing your intention on anything with laser like precision, you can make it your reality. If you live your life in fear, chances are very good you'll find something very tangible, like a cancer, to be afraid of. You already know about placebo effect, or spontaneous healing, when patients merely believe they are cured, they are. And those who believe they are not, are not. It's not the pill, it's their belief that is the key to their recovery. So what do you believe? What do you choose to experience NOW? WOW!

What marks genius is the sudden feeling of "WOW!" What every genius has said throughout history … was the same thing. "WOW!"

David Hawkins

Chapter 13

Rediscover

The Real You

Our deepest wishes are whispers of our authentic selves. We must learn to respect them. We must learn to listen.

Sarah Ban Breathnach

When the study came out about Prempro in 2002, I decided to stop taking my estrogen. My physician agreed and said I would probably experience hot flashes for a few months, and then I would be fine. The hot flashes started and stayed! I did not sleep well and was tired all the time. I became emotional over everything. I cried very easily, was anxious, and felt like I wanted to jump out of my skin. I was then referred to a reproductive endocrinologist, a gift from God I really believe. I began individualized natural biologically identical hormone replacement therapy. I have my life back! I now feel a spiritual connection in my life. The more time I take to enrich the spiritual part of my life, the more my focus is on all of the blessings I have each day. The more I take time to be in the moment, the more joy I see in the small pleasures of the day.

Judith

LIFE'S BALANCE: THE YIN AND YANG

Eastern medicine has taught for centuries that as humans, we are spiritual energy beings in a physical form. The more I practice medicine, the more I tend to agree with this ancient wisdom. The vital life force energy of our bodies, called Chi, travels via channels (meridians) to major energy centers (chakras) along your spine. Interestingly enough, these chakras correlate to some of our major organs.

Eastern medicine teaches that disturbances or blockages of this flow of universal consciousness, this Chi energy throughout our body, will result in imbalance, or dis-ease. Life is about maintaining balance of the yin (female) and the yang (male) energies in each chakra throughout our body. And the chakras correlate to your body's major organs. For instance, within the heart chakra, you have your heart, your breasts, your lungs, your shoulders, and your arms. Here's where it gets interesting to me, because you already know, the researcher in me observes and takes note of possible connections. You're well aware that type-A men have a higher risk of developing heart attacks. I believe it is very possible that this is indicative of an excess of the yang energy in the heart chakra. In contrast, women outnumber men for breast cancer development one hundred to one.

Could breast cancer represent an extreme of the yin energy in the heart chakra? Maybe. I'm open to the possibility.

IS LIFE REALLY THAT SIMPLE?

Many years ago I asked "is life simply a balance of the male/female energies in each chakra?" A few days later a new patient, aged 46, who inquired about possible choices in the management of her menopausal symptoms, gave me an answer to this question.

I started our appointment by asking how long she'd had her menopausal symptoms. After replying two years, she then told me that her symptoms had started at the time of her father's death. She went on to relate how extremely close she and her dad were, "as close as a father and daughter could possibly be". When he died, she said, her "heart broke." She then added, "In the six weeks after his death, on two separate occasions, I went out and broke an arm."

Life is about balance. Here she had her heart broken when her dad died, and then she went out and broke each of her arms separately within six weeks of his death. The arms, like the heart and breasts, also are in the heart chakra. This patient was my angel, my messenger, who informed me that life really is that simple; life is about balance of the male and female energies within each of our energy centers of our bodies.

Find something that gives you joy in life and pursue it passionately. Get out of your self and into others. Do something kind and thoughtful every day, and you'll feel your soul.

Gracelyn

MY JOURNEY TO MYSELF

As a medical physician and researcher, I used to think that I was my brain, my mind, that logical, rational, practical human being. Then, on August 21, 1983, at my father's death, I had the ultimate human experience. I went into the afterlife with my father as he passed.

My Dad was a simple man. He had one rule, the Golden Rule: Do unto others as you would have them do unto you. I never heard him speak an unkind word to or about anyone. He was a compassionate, caring man with a fantastic sense of family and he loved to laugh. Dad thought life was a whole lot of fun.

In Oprah Winfrey's book "What I Know For Sure," she says "I often wonder what Steve Jobs saw when he uttered his last words: *Oh, wow. Oh, wow. Oh, wow.*"

I was with my father when he passed so I know what Steve Jobs experienced. It is definitionless awareness, simple and nonjudgmental.

 In that space between thoughts, there is nothing to see, nothing to hear, nothing to touch, nothing to smell, nothing to taste. There is just Being. There is no time and no space. The apparent emptiness or void is filled with Infinite, Unconditional, Divine Love, Joy, Inner Peace, Bliss, Appreciation, Gratitude, and Grace.

I believe that human beings are placed on earth to love each other, to seek inner peace and happiness, as we are being of service to All That Is, including your Self. I believe that all humans have the ability to discover their own true Self, regardless of their cultural or religious background. You, too, have the ability to discover your true Self, to awaken from the illusion of the endless daily ego-motivated dramas, traumas, delusions and minutia. The beauty of awareness is that as you become true to your Self, doors will begin to open to you that you never dreamed possible. Once this door is opened it can never be closed. As you remain on your path and follow your passion, you will find that your life flows effortlessly.

Once you let go of the "should haves," "could haves," or "would haves," you begin to discover your true Self.

We all create our own perception of who we think we are. You say to yourself, "I can do this, but I can't do that". This is the box that we build. But perception is not necessarily reality. This is a mind thing; it is not real, and like most of our life experiences, it is an illusion based on of preconceived beliefs. This is not really who we are, this is just who we think we were. Let me ask you a question. Stop and listen to the dialogue and busyness of your mind chatter. Observe your thoughts for a moment, then ask "who is the observer behind the thoughts?" It is time to awaken. Choose to think differently. Choose to feel. Choose to know. Create a new and improved you by dis-creating the self-limiting barriers you or your parents, teachers, religion, society, government, and others have previously created for you, even though you might have swallowed their beliefs hook, line, and sinker in the past.

The beauty and wisdom of menopause and midlife is that you will begin to appreciate that you are even more beautiful, wiser, more whole, more complete, more at ONE with All That Is than you could ever dream or imagine. You are maturing, and awakening to the real you—your true Self.

I encourage you to go with the flow of life's energy. Stop paddling upstream. Only you can choose to change you. Are you over the need to do it your way, the need to control yourself, everyone and everything?

No? What a waste of life's precious energy! Surrender! Enjoy the journey down the river of life with its natural ebb and flow. Explore. Test the waters. Eventually you will know that you are here to love and be of service to yourself, to mankind and to All That Is.

Embrace every experience of every day, especially the emotions of your menopausal transition. They are trying to tell you something. Emotions flow from your essence, from your core, from your heart and soul. Emotions are indicators of our state of being in the present moment. When peaks and valleys of emotion are experienced, they let you know that something is off, out of balance, that something is not in alignment, that you are not being honest with your Self. Help create balance and harmony on the Earth now. Be courageous and take this time in your life to adopt the affirmation, Me No Pause for Menopause. Don't let menopause slow you down from being the newest and best version of you.

Me No Pause: Awaken and Empower your Self.

ACKNOWLEDGEMENTS

I thank my parents, Malachi Edward Quigley and Mary Louise Wintermeyer for their unconditional love and compassion, as well as their willingness to allow me to explore my life, my way. I thank my three sisters, Caroline, Meg and Therese, and my three brothers, John, Patrick, and Dan for their constant love and support in everything I have ever done. I would also like thank:

Dr. Kinch for asking me, "Have you ever thought of medicine?"

Dr. James and Therese Wiley for inviting me to Ottawa for a week to see "what medicine was really like".

Dean Bocking and the University of Western Ontario Medical School for having the confidence in me and allowing me into medical school despite less than stellar grades during my first two years of college. Drs. Hugh Allen, John Collins, Ralph Anderson, Earl Plunkett and others in the Department of Obstetrics and Gynecology at the University Western Ontario for their example, patience, and dedication to allow me to be the best clinician I could be.

Dr. Samuel Yen, who allowed me to visualize academic medicine from the top and gave me the freedom to explore whatever intrigued me at the moment in psycho-neuroendocrinology: the study of the interaction between hormones, the brain, and behavior. Every day was Christmas.

Dr. Purvis Martin, who was the perfect gentleman and scholar, and who trusted me with his treasured menopausal practice so I could set out and seek the truth about menopause from the patients themselves. Every day was Thanksgiving Day.

My partners at the IGO Medical Group in San Diego who have allowed me to function outside Western medicine's box to assist those who sought my help; and the nurses and staff at IGO for their constant support.

And my patients! Thank you for sharing your worst and best moments. Thank you for being the perfect students and teachers. Each of you make up a portion of my viewpoint about the role of estrogen and testosterone and progesterone in the reversal of menopausal symptoms. Know that you can awaken to your newest and most improved you; much wiser, energized and ready to assist in the current transition from a Patriarchal to a Matriarchal society, where we do what we do out of love and compassion, rather than out of fear or for money, power or sex.

Peter Economy and Henry Covey for the patience and willingness to review 200 plus PowerPoint slides and a mountain of information.

Danny Pietryk and Dr. Denis Bedat for their support in helping me with one of my life's missions, "to write the book."

All of the women who have read the various revisions of my book and given me their honest, constructive feedback.

Finally I wish to thank Lori Stoddard and Cory Quigley for their love, wisdom, kindness, dedication and perseverance to simplify my "doctor and researcher" version of the book so millions of women could appreciate that individualized, bio-identical, non-oral estrogen, testosterone and progesterone may be a safe and effective means of restoring their quality of life.

This book is dedicated to my three daughters, Katie, Megan and Cory; to my four granddaughters, Addison, Karly, Scarlett and Kennedy; to my grandson, Levi; and to my future grandchildren and great-grandchildren.

To learn more about women's health and how you can be a part of our global initiative of Wellness, Oneness, and Wholeness, please visit our website at quigleyfoundation.com.

The Quigley Foundation is a non-profit corporation dedicated to improving the health and wellness of women, men and their families everywhere.

Medical Disclaimer

This book offers health, fitness and nutritional information and is designed for educational purposes only. You should consult your physician or other health care professional before starting this or any other health/wellness program to determine if it is right for your needs. You should not rely on this information as a substitute for, nor does it replace, professional medical advice, diagnosis, or treatment. If you have any concerns or questions about your health, you should always consult with a physician or other health-care professional. Do not disregard, avoid or delay obtaining medical or health related advice from your health-care professional because of something you may have read in this book. The use of any information provided in this book is solely at your own risk.

Developments in medical research may impact the health, fitness and nutritional advice that appears here. No assurance can be given that the advice contained in this book will always include the most recent findings or developments with respect to the particular material.